Taiwan, Humanitarianism and Global Governance

In this unique book, Alain Guilloux uses four major elements of governance – namely norms, actors, processes and outcomes – to examine Taiwan's national governance as well as its participation in global governance in relation to humanitarian aid.

Including case studies on Taiwan's application to become an observer to the WHO, and its foreign-aid policy and practice dealing with disease outbreaks and natural disasters, Guilloux explores the complexities and dilemmas of providing humanitarian aid to people in need and distress. Taking into account Taiwan's unclear status in the global arena, and how in its efforts Taiwan faces both international isolation and opposition from the People's Republic of China at multiple levels.

Taiwan, Humanitarianism and Global Governance will be of interest for scholars of Chinese studies, Taiwan Studies, East Asian politics and International Relations, and environmental politics and humanitarian studies.

Alain Guilloux gained a PhD in political science from the University of Hong Kong in 2007. He is a former executive, board member and member of the international council of Médecins Sans Frontières and works as a researcher, consultant, writer and speaker on humanitarian and governance issues.

Routledge Research on Taiwan

Series Editor: Dafydd Fell
SOAS, UK

The *Routledge Research on Taiwan Series* seeks to publish quality research on all aspects of Taiwan studies. Taking an interdisciplinary approach, the books will cover topics such as politics, economic development, culture, society, anthropology and history.

This new book series will include the best possible scholarship from the social sciences and the humanities and welcomes submissions from established authors in the field as well as from younger authors. In addition to research monographs and edited volumes general works or textbooks with a broader appeal will be considered.

The Series is advised by an international Editorial Board and edited by Dafydd Fell of the Centre of Taiwan Studies at the School of Oriental and African Studies.

1 **Taiwan, Humanitarianism and Global Governance**
Alain Guilloux

Taiwan, Humanitarianism and Global Governance

Alain Guilloux

Routledge
Taylor & Francis Group
LONDON AND NEW YORK

First published 2009
by Routledge
2 Park Square, Milton Park, Abingdon, Oxon OX14 4RN

Simultaneously published in the USA and Canada
by Routledge
711 Third Avenue, New York, NY 10017

Routledge is an imprint of the Taylor & Francis Group, an informa business

First issued in paperback 2013

Typeset in Times by Wearset Ltd, Boldon, Tyne and Wear

British Library Cataloguing in Publication Data
A catalogue record for this book is available from the British Library

Library of Congress Cataloging-in-Publication Data
Guilloux, Alain.
Taiwan, humanitarianism and global governance/Alain Guilloux.
p. cm. – (Routledge research on Taiwan)
1. Humanitarian assistance, Taiwanese. 2. World Health Organization.
3. Taiwan–Relations–Foreign countries. I. Title.
HV555.T28.G85 2009
338.91'51249–dc22
2008043455

ISBN13: 978-0-415-46953-1 (hbk)
ISBN13: 978-0-203-87965-8 (ebk)
ISBN13: 978-0-415-66596-4 (pbk)

To Beena, Sophie, Satchet and my parents.
To François Jean and Marcel Roux

Contents

Foreword x
Acknowledgements xii
List of abbreviations xiv

1 Introduction 1

Focus of study 1
Overview of analytical framework 2
Research questions, hypotheses and associated issues 3
Case studies and data collection 4
Chapter overview 5

2 Analytical framework: states and governance 9

Introduction 9
Multiple meanings, uses and bases of 'governance' 9
States in context 13
Governance discourse and systems 17
Governance in the global context 25
Governance in the context of humanitarian action 28
Analytical framework: a summary 33

3 Taiwan: state, governance and society in perspective 35

Introduction 35
An irregular state 35
State–society interactions 43
How the state mobilizes non-state actors in external relations 48
Concluding comments 51

4 Taiwan's WHO campaign: key governance elements 53

Introduction 53
Governance norms: the WHO and Taiwan's bid for observer status 54
Governance actors: the WHO and Taiwan's bid for observer status 61
Governance processes: the WHO and Taiwan's bid for observer status 68
Governance outputs and outcomes: the WHO and Taiwan's bid for observer status 76
Concluding comments and questions 78

5 Taiwan's WHO campaign: discussion 80

Introduction 80
Governance norms revisited 80
Governance actors revisited 91
Governance processes revisited 95
Governance outputs and outcomes revisited 98
Concluding comments and questions 105

6 Taiwan's medical and humanitarian aid experience: key governance elements 107

Introduction 107
Governance norms 107
Governance actors 112
Governance processes 117
Governance outputs and outcomes 126
Concluding comments and questions 134

7 Taiwan's medical and humanitarian aid experience: discussion 135

Introduction 135
Governance norms revisited 135
Governance actors revisited 141
Governance processes revisited 147
Governance outputs and outcomes revisited 152
Concluding comments 163

8 Conclusion: a revisiting 165

Research questions and hypotheses revisited 165
Case analyses revisited 166
Taiwan and irregular states revisited 171
Governance and governance theory revisited 175

References 179
Index 199

Foreword

Governance is a versatile phenomenon of considerable significance in many areas of public and private life. It is capable, at one and the same time, of embracing both macro-level patterns of inter-institutional engagement and micro-level modes of intra-institutional operation. This kind of application at contrasting levels can be relevant not only within the one context in each case, but also across contexts, be they local, national or international. The result is a diverse array of institutional arrangements whose foundations, work and achievements are the consequences of some form of governance thinking and action.

This book recognizes the scope and value of governance – as a theoretical construct and a practical reality. The construct gives rise to an analytical framework which is used to address the reality of Taiwan's moves to join the World Health Organization and to provide international medical and humanitarian assistance in the service of enhancing its reputation and standing in the international community. The framework is comprehensive and compelling, as are the case discussions from which numerous insights are gained and lessons learnt about the power, politics and policy initiatives involved.

The framework established is sound testimony to the reach of governance theory. Global forces and developments justify its inclusion of selected theories of international relations, along with political systems theory and regime theory. This broad conception of governance is appropriately accompanied by a more specific concentration on norms and values, actors and related entities, processes and instruments, and outputs and outcomes. These aspects of governance, mostly informed by policy theories and models, complement global interests and concerns, while sharpening the focus on particular strategies which states can, and do, adopt in pursuit of national and international objectives.

The Taiwan context is particularly interesting and raises questions of governance, power and politics that are not necessarily relevant, or as relevant, in other contexts. An underlying argument is that Taiwan is an 'irregular' state with motivations and goals often not matched by 'regular' states. Its 'irregularity' has had an impact on much of its international activity, including its initiatives concerning the WHO and international medical and humanitarian assistance.

The detailed discussions of Taiwan's experience in these two areas confirm the utility of case study methodology. The stories told are enlightening and telling in ways usually only best informed by case analyses.

The book has much to commend to it. It makes a significant contribution to governance knowledge and understanding, with a challenge to others to examine both 'irregular' and 'regular' states as consciously strategic actors in the global arena.

Ian Thynne
Charles Darwin University
Australia

Acknowledgements

First of all I would like to express my gratitude to Ian Thynne, my primary supervisor and a former Visiting Professor at the Department of Politics and Public Administration of the University of Hong Kong. From him I learnt a lot about methods and governance theory through numerous and cheerful exchanges, structured discussions and detailed e-mails. Above all, I deeply appreciated his continued commitment and support after he left for Darwin. James Tang supported me at key stages of my research and I benefited from his insights as well as his numerous invitations to participate in conferences, seminars and symposiums. I also benefited from exchanges with many others at the department including Sonny Loh, Irene Tong, Joseph Chan, Danny Lam, Peter Cheung, Ken Wang, Lucy Cummings, Maria Francesch and Rikkie Yeung. Miron Mushkat was a stimulating and challenging guide through the numerous traps of research methods. I am also grateful to John Burns and Guy Peters for testing my ability to clarify key ideas at the final stage.

At the Centre of Asian Studies, I benefited from discussions with Wong Siu-lun, Nick Thomas, Isabelle Saint-Mézard and Prakash Metaparti and from the opportunity to present my ideas at a workshop on regionalism and governance.

I would also like to thank the University of Hong Kong's Committee on Research and Conference Grants for a travel grant that made field research in Geneva and Paris possible, and the *Centre d'Etudes Français sur la Chine Contemporaine* (CEFC) for a travel grant to Taiwan. In addition, I benefited from many informal discussions with Gilles Guiheux.

At WHO headquarters in Geneva many people who prefer, understandably, to remain anonymous were of help and assisted me in many ways, with valuable contacts and information. Daniel Tang was very effective in organizing contacts and interviews at TaiwanICDF and the Ministry of Foreign Affairs. Peter Chang gave me the opportunity to discuss some of my ideas in a forum with aid officials and NGOs in Taipei. By e-mail and on the phone Yan-di Chang shared her experience and pointed out invaluable resources. My heartfelt thanks to all of them for their help.

I am indebted to Rony Brauman for his many insights, shared during discussions that started long before I set out to work on this research, on all aspects of humanitarian aid and in particular the many ways in which states use disaster relief activities, humanitarian symbols and organizations to advance their own interests. The same goes for many others at Médecins sans Frontières, in particular the late François Jean and Marcel Roux.

Finally, but most importantly, I would like to thank my wife Beena Sorab for her patience, unflinching support and encouragements throughout these years.

List of abbreviations

ADB	Asian Development Bank
ANC	African National Congress
APEC	Asia-Pacific Economic Cooperation
ASEAN	Association of Southeast Asian Nations
BLIA	Buddha's Light International Association
CABEI	Central American Bank for Economic Integration
CARES	Chinese Association for Relief and Ensuing Services
CCM	Country-Coordinating Mechanism
CDC	Centre for Disease Control
CMH	Commission on Macroeconomic and Health
CoA	Council of Agriculture
CSI	Civil Society Initiative
CSO	Civil Society Organization
CTC	Congressional Taiwan Caucus
DAC	Development Assistance Committee
DfID	Department for International Development
DIO	Department of International Organizations
DNDi	Drugs for Neglected Diseases initiative
DoH	Taiwan Department of Health
DPO	Department of Peacekeeping Operations
DPP	Democratic Progressive Party
DPU	Democratic Pacific Union
EBRD	European Bank for Reconstruction and Development
ECHO	European Community Humanitarian Office
ECOSOC	Economic and Social Council of the United Nations
ECOWAS	Economic Community of West African States
EU	European Union
EV71	Enterovirus 71
FAPA	Formosan Association for Public Affairs
FDI	Foreign Direct Investment
FMPAT	Foundation of Medical Professionals Alliance in Taiwan
GATT	General Agreement on Tariffs and Trade
GBC	Global Business Coalition

GDP	Gross Domestic Product
GHI	Global Health Initiative
GIO	Government Information Office
GNI	Gross National Income
GOARN	Global Outbreak Alert and Response Network
GPG	Global Public Good
GPPP	Global Public–Private Partnership
GPPPH	Global Public–Private Partnership for Health
GTZ	Deutsche Gesellschaft für Technische Zusammenarbeit [German Agency for Technical Cooperation]
HAJCO	Hashemite Jordan Charity Organization
HDI	Human Development Index
HFMD	Hand, Foot and Mouth Disease
iACT	International Action and Cooperation Team
ICH	International Conference on Harmonization of Technical Requirements for Registration of Pharmaceuticals for Human Use
ICBL	International Campaign to Ban Landmines
ICN	International Council of Nursing
ICRC	International Committee of the Red Cross
ICU	International Cooperation Unit, Taiwan Department of Health
IDA	International Development Association
IECDF	International Economic Cooperation Development Fund (Taiwan)
IFC	International Finance Corporation
IFPMA	International Federation of Pharmaceutical Manufacturers & Associations
IFRC	International Federation of Red Cross and Red Crescent Societies
IGO	Intergovernmental Organization
IHR	International Health Regulations
IHRF	International Humanitarian Relief Fund (Taiwan)
ILO	International Labour Organization
IMF	International Monetary Fund
INGO	International Non-governmental Organization
IP	Intellectual Property
IPA	International Paediatrics Association
IPF	International Pharmaceutical Federation
IRC	International Rescue Committee
ISI	Import-Substitution Industrialization
KMT	Kuo Ming Tang
LDCs	Least Developed Countries
LIBOR	London Inter Bank Offering Rate
LICs	Low-Income Countries
MDGs	Millennium Development Goals
MDM	Médecins du Monde

MDRTB	Multidrug Resistant Tuberculosis
MMV	Medicines for Malaria Venture
MNC	Multinational Corporation
MoFA	Ministry of Foreign Affairs
MSF	Médecins Sans Frontières
NAFTA	North American Free Trade Agreement
NATO	North Atlantic Treaty Organization
NGO	Non-Governmental Organization
NPO	Non-Profit Organization
ODA	Official Development Assistance
OECD	Organization for Economic Cooperation and Development
OIHP	Office International d'Hygiène Publique [International Office of Public Hygiene]
PLO	Palestine Liberation Organization
PRC	Peoples' Republic of China
ROC	Republic of China
SAR	Special Administrative Region
SARS	Severe Acute Respiratory Syndrome
SME	Small and Medium-sized Enterprise
SOE	State-Owned Enterprise
TaiwanICDF	International Cooperation and Development Fund (Taiwan)
TaiwanIHA	Taiwan International Health Alliance
TB	Tuberculosis
TDR	Tropical Disease Research
TIMA	Taiwan International Medical Alliance
TNA	Transnational Advocacy Network
TNC	Transnational Corporation
TOAID	Taiwan Overseas Aid and International Development Alliance
TOPS	Taipei Overseas Peace Services
TRIPS	Trade-Related Aspects of Intellectual Property Rights
TRMPC	Taiwan Roots Medical Peace Corps
UN	United Nations
UNDP	United Nations Development Programme
UNDPI	United Nations Department of Public Information
UNESCO	United Nations Educational, Scientific and Cultural Organization
UNFPA	United Nations Population Fund
UNHCR	United Nations High Commissioner for Refugees
UNICEF	United Nations Children's Fund
UNOCHA	United Nations Office for the Coordination of Humanitarian Affairs
UNODC	United Nations Office on Drugs and Crime
UNPO	Unrepresented Nations and Peoples Organization
UNSC	United Nations Security Council
USAID	United States Agency for International Development
WFP	World Food Programme

WHA	World Health Assembly
WHO	World Health Organization
WHPA	World Health Professionals Alliance
WMA	World Medical Association
WTO	World Trade Organization

1 Introduction

Focus of study

This study addresses Taiwan's involvement in important aspects of the global order or arena from a state-centred governance perspective. Taiwan has long been regarded as an irregular state. On the one hand it enjoys limited, low international recognition. On the other, it has become an economic and trading powerhouse and is a key link in the global technology production system. In addition, it has had a remarkably successful and smooth democratic transition. But as it struggles for recognition, Taiwan does not have access to the whole range of options normally open to states that enjoy international recognition. At the same time, its successful political evolution and impressive economic achievements provide Taiwan with a range of options that may not be available to many other countries – especially developing ones.

Over the last two decades Taiwan has become a provider of technical, economic and humanitarian aid. Other countries or territories in East Asia, including Hong Kong and Singapore, have also become significant aid providers over the same period. Hong Kong has a vibrant sector in terms of non-state aid organizations, but the input of the government remains weak. Conversely, in Singapore the response of the state has been stronger, but non-state actors have had a very limited role in responding to crises overseas. Focusing on Taiwan seems more interesting, as both state and non-state actors and organizations have been quite active. It is therefore expected that a wider range of interactions between state and non-state actors will be observed in Taiwan.

Taiwan's aid programmes have long been dismissed by their critics as 'dollar diplomacy', which refers to the purchase of diplomatic alliances through gifts of various kinds. Does this set Taiwan apart from other donors? To explore this issue, two interrelated case studies are provided to address different aspects of Taiwan's involvement in the global response system to life-threatening crises: public health crises and the response to natural and man-made disasters. The first case study considers Taiwan's campaign to gain observer status at the World Health Assembly/World Health Organization. The second case study explores Taiwan's contribution to life-saving goals through medical and humanitarian aid programmes.

Overview of analytical framework

To explore these issues, an analytical framework is developed in Chapter 2 with reference to state-centred activity and ideas about governance. The state is the key driver of governance processes as it represents, at least in democratic political systems, the legitimate aspirations of citizens. At the same time, the state interacts in many ways with the market and civil society through its various organizations.

Governance implies numerous interrelationships between or among the state, market and civil society in which various people and organizations, as players or actors, are central elements. Governance is a complex, multidimensional phenomenon. As a concept or set of ideas, it assists effectively in making sense of the ways in which states, markets and civil societies interact, both domestically and internationally, in the formulation and implementation of policies for collective purposes and causes.

Governance is understood here as a system comprising four directly interrelated elements:

- norms in the form of widely expected modes of behaviour and associated values and principles;
- actors in terms of people and organizations of the state, market and civil society;
- processes including linking arrangements and policy tools or instruments; and
- outputs and outcomes in terms of achievements and their impact or effect.

These elements have been addressed in other lines of theory, in particular regime theory, political systems theory, institutionalism and various streams of IR theory. The emphasis may be on one of these elements or on a specific set of elements. Some authors argue that what primarily matters is for everyone to follow certain norms. Others point to the decisive role of specific actors. Others again mainly focus on the processes involved. Lastly, the end result is the primary concern of some researchers.

The governance framework builds on these other theories. All four elements are significant and useful in understanding how governance works. The governance framework valuably integrates them to provide an understanding of the structures and processes associated with governing. In practice, the elements may interact in a variety of ways. Actors may be influenced by certain norms, while also competing for influence over norm-setting. The emergence of new norms may lead to the creation and involvement of new actors. Norms may strongly influence processes, if potential actors are to agree on the way processes will be driven. Actors obviously influence, and are selective in, the processes utilized. The activities of actors in and through various processes result in outputs and outcomes.

These interrelationships constitute a sound basis on which to describe and assess how the various features of a state and governance system influence one another and how, in accordance with existing norms, some actors agree on a set of processes to deliver specific outputs or achieve specific outcomes. Together, they assist valuably in exploring and making sense of Taiwan's involvement in the global arena and more specifically in the healthcare and humanitarian fields.

Research questions, hypotheses and associated issues

The ideas about states and governance outlined here and developed in detail in Chapter 2 suggest various research questions about Taiwan's health and humanitarian initiatives in the global arena. The questions, in turn, lead to various general hypotheses about the nature and extent of that experience.

Key sets of questions include the following:

- In what ways does Taiwan involve itself in the global arena in response to public health issues and natural or man-made disasters? Are the ways always consciously designed to enhance its status in the global arena?
- Does Taiwan use all, or only some, of the elements of governance in this field? In the process, in what ways does it link up with the actors most likely to support it?
- Does Taiwan use the elements of governance in ways that are different from those of other states? If so, does it refer to norms other states do not usually emphasize? Also, does it involve itself with a different set of organizations and processes?

The key hypotheses are:

- Taiwan has a definite need strategically to use all of the elements of governance at its disposal to facilitate its involvement in the global arena.
- Taiwan uses the elements of governance in ways which differ significantly from those of other states.
- Taiwan forms alliances with other governance actors in ways which differ significantly from those formed by other states.

Also of interest are the dynamics or evolution of a given system of governance over time. If specific outputs or outcomes are regarded as unsatisfactory, norms may evolve, some actors may withdraw, new actors may join in, and processes may be modified. Repeated observations help make sense of the bigger picture, taking into account changes in norms and processes and in the distribution of power between relevant actors.

In national governance, the primacy of the state and the principle of sovereignty point to a hierarchy of norms and actors. Sovereignty remains the key principle and the state remains the core actor even after many iterations of the governance cycle, unless the state disappears, is challenged by violent internal conflict, or is deemed a threat to international peace. In contrast, no similar hierarchy exists in the global arena, as the international system is characterized by anarchy and no actor can claim sovereignty over all the others. Competing or conflicting norms and legitimacies are therefore a key feature of global governance.

These issues lead to a more general set of research questions. If participants in a governance system are pursuing not just the common good but also particular interests, what will be the impact on the system? In what ways will the dynamic, architecture and characteristics of the system be affected? What is the evolution of a global system over time?

It is likely that coalitions of actors of various types will form around key issues on the basis of shared interests. It is also likely that a system that delivers outputs and outcomes in line with the expectations of relevant actors will remain stable over time; or conversely, where actors are divided or dissatisfied, the governance system will be forced to change.

Case studies and data collection

The questions, hypotheses and issues raised here are explored through two case studies of Taiwan's involvement in the global response system to life-threatening situations: public health crises and the response to natural and man-made disasters. The two case studies focus on the ways in which Taiwan uses the elements of governance to advance its own interests.

The first case study focuses on Taiwan's campaign to gain observer status at the World Health Organization (WHO) and therefore emphasizes Taiwan's goal to achieve international recognition through addressing significant public health issues. The second case study explores Taiwan's contribution to life-saving goals through overseas medical and humanitarian assistance.

The two case studies are interrelated. Taiwan's medical and humanitarian aid activities are one of the components of the WHO campaign. These programmes also constitute part of Taiwan's efforts to retain or win official diplomatic allies. Such diplomatic alliances in turn help Taiwan in its WHO campaign.

In the WHO case study, such observations are made over the period since the campaign started. In particular, outcomes are observed at regular intervals, as the World Health Assembly is held every year in May. Taiwan's contribution to medical and humanitarian aid programmes developed gradually and was very limited until the 1990s.

Data were collected both from primary and secondary sources. Primary sources include information about the various organizations involved, their mandates, missions, structure, activities and programmes. Such information was collected from the documents published by these organizations in print and on their websites.

Primary sources also include unstructured interviews conducted during field-studies in Taiwan, Geneva and Paris. In particular, interviews were conducted with WHO executives, Taiwanese officials, Taiwanese NGOs and international NGOs. In addition, extensive and informative exchanges by e-mail and telephone with Yan-Di Chang in New York must be mentioned.

Data were also collected from secondary sources, mostly print and electronic media. In addition, a significant amount of data regarding Taiwanese NGOs was collected from a survey of Taiwanese humanitarian organizations carried out by Taiwan International Medical Alliance (2004).

Chapter overview

The analytical framework of the thesis is developed in Chapter 2, with the key focus on the interactions of states and governance. While states are both providers and consumers of governance discourses, symbols and systems, they do not control all of them. This leads to a complex pattern of interrelationships between the state, market and civil society. While each of these spheres has its own legitimacy and relative autonomy, the state remains the central actor in the system. Governance is a multidimensional concept which helps make sense of these interactions, both domestically and internationally. It comprises four interrelated elements, as indicated in the analytical overview provided above.

The ideas and elements of governance are, first, addressed in general. Governance emphasizes the idea that the market and civil society can be enrolled along with the state in the provision of public goods, which is seen as positive not just in terms of resource mobilization but also of enhanced legitimacy. These ideas and elements are then reframed in the context of global governance. While states invoke norms, use organizations and manipulate processes to achieve specific outputs and outcomes, their actions may be questioned by both domestic and external forces in the global context.

The elements of governance are then applied specifically to humanitarian action, although the set of arrangements designed to respond to life-threatening emergencies is driven by many motives other than humanitarian. The tension between humanitarian and political motives is highlighted. The discussion addresses the various governance actors, processes, outputs and outcomes applied more specifically to the sphere of humanitarian action and the ways in which states can use humanitarian issues for significant domestic purposes and to advance their position in international relations.

Taiwan's state and society are introduced in Chapter 3. The focus here is not on evaluating Taiwan's claim to statehood, but on Taiwan's disputed, irregular status, the island's troubled history and its specific location on the map of political entities: what is Taiwan? The discussion is in particular centred on Taiwan's involvement in the global arena, its limited diplomatic recognition and the obstacles to its participation in intergovernmental organizations.

As Taiwan was often described as a strong developmental state, the evolution of state–society relations and linkages is highlighted throughout the phases of Taiwan's democratization. How far does the strong state paradigm help explain Taiwan's evolution? How effectively did non-state actors contribute to Taiwan's successful development from a poor territory under siege to an economic and trading powerhouse and a vibrant democracy? The respective contributions of the state and society are highlighted.

This leads to an overview of the involvement of non-state actors in Taiwan's external relations. As Taiwan reached an all-time low in external recognition in the 1980s, a new policy, labelled pragmatic diplomacy, was implemented after Taiwan started moving towards full-fledged democratization. In particular, pragmatic diplomacy rested on informal contacts, including the increased involvement of Taiwanese non-state organizations, both for-profit and non-profit, in external relations. The characteristics of this policy are highlighted and its achievements discussed, in particular with regard to the NGO Affairs Committee set up by the government and its focus on increasing the participation of Taiwanese NGOs in international NGOs and their exposure to UN institutions. More widely, the identity issue is linked to the unclear status of Taiwan and the island's democratization. The chapter sets the scene for the two case studies.

Chapter 4 introduces the key governance elements relevant to Taiwan's bid to become an observer at the World Health Organization. The bid is analysed here in terms of the categories identified in Chapter 2 as key elements of governance: norms, actors, processes, both in terms of linking arrangements between the participants and the policy instruments they use, outputs and outcomes. The elements are identified with regard to the WHO in general following an overview of international medical cooperation since the 1850s. The same governance elements are used to introduce, in parallel, Taiwan's campaign to obtain observer status. In particular, Taiwan refers to three sets of norms – political, scientific/medical/technical and humanitarian – which also structure the WHO's mandate. An important point is that these norms can be invoked and used in combination to enhance their effectiveness.

The input of market and civil society organizations in Taiwan's bid also mirrors the input of the same types of actors in the WHO's activities. While the status of members and associate members is clearly defined in the WHO's constitution, uncertainty and flexibility characterize observer status. Taiwan's bid therefore generates uncertainty over Taiwan's ultimate goal. As Taiwan is an irregular state, attention is paid in particular to the specific issues that make its bid problematic.

In Chapter 5 the elements of governance systems are brought together to provide a more comprehensive analysis and discussion of the campaign. The first set of issues relates to governance norms. Are Taiwan's arguments relevant and its invocation of political, medical and humanitarian norms credible? The focus is here on the validity of the arguments and the ways in which political, humanitarian and medical norms are combined. Another set of issues relates to the identity and nature of the governance actors involved in Taiwan's campaign. In the light of the findings and discussion of Chapter 3, is it possible to categorize these actors clearly? Or is the division between state and non-state organizations unclear if not blurred?

A third set of issues relates to governance processes. What are the patterns of interaction between the organizations involved in Taiwan's bid? One area of particular interest is the degree of insertion of Taiwan in the WHO's relevant governance processes both through state and non-state actors. Another area of interest is the way Taiwanese authorities use the mix of policy instruments at their disposal. Lastly, it is interesting to assess Taiwan's strategy in terms of outputs and outcomes. If Taiwan's objective is to be admitted as an observer at the World Health Assembly, is the output appropriate? Alternatively, Taiwan may have other objectives in mind. Possible outcomes of the campaign, whether intended or unintended, are examined here.

In Chapter 6 the focus is on the humanitarian and medical aid provided by Taiwanese organizations to overseas countries or territories. The governance elements of norms, actors, processes, outputs and outcomes are again being used to structure and inform the discussion of the humanitarian and medical aid provided by Taiwan, in parallel with that of global actors. As in the case of Taiwan's WHO campaign, there are political, scientific/medical/technical and humanitarian dimensions to Taiwan's aid. In addition to these three dimensions already introduced in Chapters 2 and 4, economic norms and arguments are introduced here.

The rapid evolution of global health cooperation is highlighted. In the past two decades, mounting challenges and persistent dissatisfaction with global health outcomes have led to the reappraisal of existing norms, the creation of new actors including at the global level, a significant increase in both public and private resources and a commitment to measurable targets publicized as the Millennium Development Goals.

Taiwan's past and present efforts are introduced against this background. Several state institutions focus in part on the provision of medical and humanitarian assistance, in particular the Ministry of Foreign Affairs, the International Cooperation and Development Fund (TaiwanICDF) and the Council of Agriculture. Several Taiwanese NGOs have also contributed significantly through their own programmes. Other medical and humanitarian aid projects are carried out jointly by governmental and non-governmental organizations. The Taiwanese government appears eager to capitalize on all these programmes to advance its own diplomatic interests in terms of enhanced recognition in general and in particular promote its WHO bid.

These findings are discussed in Chapter 7. Key governance elements again serve as a guide to the analysis of Taiwan's medical and humanitarian aid in the broader perspective of the global aid system. The significance and dimensions of Taiwan's initiatives in the field of medical and humanitarian assistance are assessed. To what extent do state and non-state Taiwanese actors conform to rapidly evolving global norms? Do Taiwan's medical and humanitarian aid actors resemble counterparts in other donor countries? Is Taiwan's aid relevant to the outcomes Taiwan targets?

In terms of governance processes, the linking arrangements and policy instruments used by the various actors involved in Taiwan's medical and humanitarian aid are discussed here. Taiwan's unclear status and limited recognition may force the government to give more leeway to non-state actors, or in contrast make the government more dependent on these actors. Taiwanese aid actors, whether state or non-state, may face obstacles because of Taiwan's status. These issues are examined here. Lastly, it is important to look at Taiwan's aid outputs and outcomes. Do they match global expectations? Specifically, does its unclear status lead Taiwan to deliver atypical outputs or seek outcomes that it would otherwise not be interested in?

The findings and discussions are brought together in Chapter 8. Taiwan participates in the global health and disaster response systems in many ways and, in doing so, uses key elements of governance. While Taiwan refers to global norms and its programmes involve actors and organizations of all types, aid outputs and outcomes lack visibility.

Taiwan points to its various programmes and related contributions as key arguments in support of its WHO bid. But the potential of this contribution is limited as Taiwan remains an irregular state. Taiwanese aid actors operate with additional constraints due to Taiwan's international isolation.

This leads to some general conclusions with regard to the dynamics of global governance systems and their evolution over time. As actors in governance systems, first and foremost states, pursue their own interests and not just the common good, the characteristics and evolution of such systems remain fluid. In this environment, norms are important as their selective invocation allows actors to disguise their own interests and increase leverage.

Norms, actors, processes, outputs and outcomes are key elements of the framework developed in the next chapter. One of its main purposes is to assist in describing how the various elements of a governance system interact. The framework will thus help make sense of the ways governance systems function, deliver or fail to deliver, and evolve. Eventually, it is also hoped it will help provide a sound conceptual basis for new lines of theory development.

2 Analytical framework

States and governance

Introduction

This chapter develops the analytical framework of the thesis. The framework is exploratory rather than explanatory. It provides structure and content in accordance with the research questions and hypotheses set out in Chapter 1. Overall, it is a comprehensive conceptual basis for guiding and informing the discussions in subsequent empirical chapters, leading to possible new lines of theory development in the concluding chapter.

The key focus is on the interactions of states and governance. States generate, control and make use of governance discourses and systems. They also have to respond to governance discourses and systems initiated, controlled and used by others in the various arenas in which they operate.

Multiple meanings, uses and bases of 'governance'

The term 'governance' has been defined and used in multiple ways over the past decades: for example as a phenomenon, a concept, a process, a basis of collective action, and a political project/policy prescription – as appreciated, among numerous authors, by Hoffmann and Ba (2005) and Pierre and Peters (2000). It implies numerous relationships between or among individuals, groups, organizations and institutions. These relationships are forged and maintained at various levels within and beyond systems and they operate across various areas of activity. As they increasingly involve the state, market and civil society, governance inevitably embraces political, economic and social ideas, forms and issues. Its various elements can be synthesized in the form of an analytical framework, which assists effectively in making sense of the ways in which policies are formulated and action is taken for collective purposes and causes, both domestically and globally.

As a phenomenon, 'governance' primarily characterizes the role of non-state actors in policy-making and policy implementation. While the traditional approach to policy-making focused exclusively on government and state, the role of non-state actors in policy-making and policy implementation grew over the past two decades.

In the 1960s and 1970s, public choice theorists started questioning the role of the state in the delivery of public goods and services. Specifically, they questioned the claim that states' outputs automatically resulted in optimal outcomes and pointed to the negative side effects of Keynesianism, welfare and the self-serving interests of politicians and bureaucrats (Hindmoor, 2006). Increasingly, the state relied on the input of other actors, which contributed resources and provided legitimacy to its action (Pierre and Peters, 2000).

Similarly, global governance as a phenomenon highlights the increasing roles and contributions of non-state actors in decision-making and implementation with regard to global issues. In the global arena, state power is also bounded by the impact of external forces and actors, both state and non-state. Whereas the state has authority over non-state actors in a domestic setting, there is no certainty with regard to the nature of the links between actors in a global setting. Some actors may be subjected to some kind of hierarchy, while others act independently. This suggests a complex mix of hierarchical authority and networking arrangements.

Second, 'governance' is a political/ideological project. As the state was increasingly criticized, in particular because of its inefficiencies, cost, rigid bureaucracy and lack of responsiveness to societal demands, its uncontrolled growth was questioned. Instead, the prescription was to give a leading role to market forces and reform government according to market-based models. More generally, 'government was now increasingly defined not as the solution to societal problems but instead as the very root and cause of these problems' (Pierre and Peters, 2000: 2).

At the global level, the governance project can be described as twofold. On the one hand, governance equals 'good governance'. Under the initial impetus of the IMF and the World Bank, governments were urged to follow market-friendly policies, reduce budget deficits, set realistic foreign exchange rates, and liberalize foreign trade. On the other hand, once these reforms are undertaken and domestic markets are opened up to foreign goods and investors, the global governance project unfolds and becomes a strategy that displaces domestic constituencies from their traditional monopoly over policy decisions in a national setting.

Third, although governance theory may still be at a rudimentary stage, the use of 'governance' signals a novel way to think about politics (Pierre and Peters, 2000). The primary emphasis is on steering rather than imposing. This leads to privileging consensus or compromises over the strict enforcement of rules, and flexibility over rigid norms or mandates.

While political science traditionally focuses on government and the role of the state, the governance approach highlights in particular the input of non-state actors and the numerous interactions between all the actors involved in governing (Pierre and Peters, 2000). It also helps focus on the norms that underpin policy-making and the processes by which policy outcomes are achieved. This broad understanding of the concept of governance goes beyond the traditional focus of comparative politics on the inputs and related elements of the governing process.

One problem with such a broad concept is that it carries a great diversity of meanings, depending on the perspectives from which it is approached. Among these perspectives, Pierre and Peters (2000) identify in particular traditional authority, autopoesis, cybernetics, policy instruments, institutional analysis, rational choice, networks and policy communities, neo-Marxism and critical theory.

Similarly, global governance has been interpreted in many different ways, given the broad range of possible meanings. Hoffmann and Ba (2005) identify nine different perspectives on global governance: international regimes; international society; hegemonic stability; dynamics of globalization; the pursuit of IMF/World Bank/UN goals; global change/global order; restructuring of the global political economy; world government; and global civil society.

A common thread between the various governance and global governance approaches is that they are all concerned with both structure and process. These aspects are explored in detail later as the analytical framework is developed.

'Governance' in its various guises has embraced various aspects of regime theory, political systems theory, institutionalism and IR theory. In essence, regime theory posits that the actors involved in governance in a particular issue-area are informed by a set of rules and norms that applies to all of them (Young, 2005). It also anticipates that these actors are likely to play by the rules and follow the norms. These actors may be state or non-state. But while regime theory recognizes the importance of rules and norms and the involvement of various types of actors and organizations, it takes a relatively static view of the governance system thus created. In particular, it does not address why a particular regime comes into being and how it may eventually give way to another. It also does not directly address the issue of the nature of global governance. Is global governance simply a collection of more or less autonomous or loosely connected regimes? Or are there elements that cut across regimes in different issue areas and provide clues regarding the architecture of global governance?

Political systems theory is founded most significantly in work by Easton (1953, 1965). It focuses on demands, supports and decision-making in political-administrative arenas in terms of the call for and acceptance of outputs in the form of policies and action. It indicates the relationships involved and the significance of feedback as a basis of policy learning, adjustment and reformulation. The relationships themselves are significant and worthy of analysis, but little is said about the actual structures of government and the state which underpin those relationships.

Issues of structure are central to institutionalism. While this approach insists that institutions matter, institutions mean different things to different theorists. Some theorists link institutions primarily to agency and culture, while others focus on legalism, hierarchy and associated developments (Hay and Lister, 2006; Schmidt, 2006). Of particular interest is the revival, over the past two decades, of studies highlighting the importance of the state as an institution with primary importance in the processes of governing (Evans *et al.*, 1985).

Different streams of IR theory have traditionally debated the importance of the state in this process. Realists insist that states are the only institutions or players that matter with regard to global governance. While they may recognize, in various measures, the increasing importance of the market, they argue that whatever power the market supposedly acquired was essentially granted with the acquiescence of the state. Global governance, in this perspective, is not expected to provide more insight than the study of interstate/intergovernmental relations, the traditional focus of IR scholars.

In contrast, liberals see the state primarily as the custodian of a wider order rooted in the individual and the rights that are naturally conferred to the citizen. As a consequence, they focus on the cooperation processes states have to enter to achieve an order compatible with these inherent rights, and on the importance of non-state actors in ensuring that states do not lose sight of the desired outcome. Liberalism as a project or policy prescription posits that as more states become liberal, international conflicts will eventually subside (Green, 2005).

Constructivists argue that power and interests can be recast as ideas (Wendt, 1999). While they insist on the importance of ideas, constructivists tend to provide a one-dimensional account of the structure of power and downplay the effects of physical power, material capabilities, and the capacity and willingness to constrain displayed by some actors.

While the various theories and approaches mentioned here provide valuable insights into important aspects of politics and governance, the actors, norms and processes of global governance cannot be reduced to any of these lines of thinking. Some scholars focus primarily on the state and therefore the role of government. Others focus on the growing importance of the market and private authority, including the dimensions of corporate governance (Fuchs, 2004; Hall and Biersteker, 2002). Others again, following a communitarian approach, insist that civil society is or should be the key actor in governance.

The focus adopted here is on state-centred governance with global significance, in recognition that the state is still (and is likely to remain for the foreseeable future) the primary instance through which citizens' preferences are processed into policy decisions. In this regard, the governance approach helps to clarify how the role of the state is transformed in a new configuration (Sorensen, 2006; Pierre and Peters, 2005). Non-state actors may constrain the state in some respects or instances. They might also act as supporters of the state, or as impact multipliers in other cases. 'The actual role which the state plays in governance is often the outcome of the tug-of-war between the role the state wants to play and the role which the external environment allows it to play' (Pierre and Peters, 2000: 26).

For the purposes of this study, governance is defined very broadly as a set of systems and processes by or through which people and organizations seek to achieve significant public goals and objectives. It comprises four interrelated elements which are especially relevant to the study:

- norms, values and principles;
- actors in terms of people and organizations;
- processes involving inter-organizational linking arrangements and policy instruments;
- outputs and outcomes.

Within the framework developed here, the characteristics of states are addressed first. The above elements of governance are then initially addressed in the context of relevant views of governance and, subsequently, of global governance. Thereafter, they are applied more specifically to the spheres of humanitarian action and the ways in which states can use humanitarian issues for significant domestic purposes or to advance their position in international relations.

States in context

Definitions and features

Weber argues that 'a compulsory political organization with continuous operations (*politischer Anstaltsbetrieb*) will be called a "state" insofar as its administrative staff successfully upholds the claims to the monopoly of the legitimate use of physical force in the enforcement of its order' (Weber, 1978: 54). A state in this regard has several features which need to be addressed.

First, a permanent institution. How to ensure that the state remains when the regime falls? Foucault argues that the state constructs its origins to establish its credentials over a long period. The state has to reinvent its past (Foucault, 1997). In reaction to the French Revolution and its invocation of universal rights, Burke invoked the rights of Englishmen, and reconstructed England on the basis of these rights (Burke, 1987). Fichte elaborated the concept of a German nation in response to the Napoleonic invasion and the invaders' insistence on imposing universal values (Fichte, 1978). China claims to be the most ancient state on earth. The harnessing of such claims and the reconstruction of history is clearly one source of state power, and reinforces its legitimacy.

Second, the monopoly of the use of force. This idea was first articulated in a comprehensive manner by Thomas Hobbes in the seventeenth century. Hobbes argued that the greatest fear of man is to be killed. As the weak can also kill the strong, the only way to achieve security is for each man to renounce his right to defend himself and transfer this natural right to the sovereign. As it is not involved in private disputes, the sovereign will protect everyone from the risk of being killed, provided all surrender their right to defend themselves (Hobbes, 1996). How do we ensure that the sovereign itself does not become a security risk to each and every one? Hobbes argues that each individual will be too insignificant to the sovereign to attract its attention, so the risk will be low. Besides, Weber argues that the monopoly is not over the exercise of violence per se, but over its legitimate exercise (Weber, 1978). The state may delegate the exercise of such legitimate violence.

Third, legitimacy. Weber argues that every system of domination 'attempts to establish and to cultivate the belief in its legitimacy' (Weber, 1978: 213) and that stability is greatest when an order 'enjoys the prestige of being considered binding, or, as it may be expressed, of "legitimacy"' (Weber, 1978: 31). What if the state's claim to legitimacy is challenged? The state can discipline the challengers and confront them with physical force: it can fine them, put them on trial, send them to prison or even execute them. Such actions may buttress the legitimacy of the state, but sometimes weaken it. Unless there is a direct and imminent threat to the country, a state may find it difficult to fully exercise its monopoly over the use of violence (such as risking soldiers' lives) and at the same time successfully uphold its claim to legitimacy. If challenged on this count, a state may declare a state of emergency, or state of exception (Schmitt, 1996). Schmitt argues that the true, ultimate nature of the state is precisely the state of exception (see also Agamben, 1999). But states may also strive to enhance legitimacy to lower the cost of extracting authority.

Fourth, territoriality. States are defined as self-governing entities with effective control over a well-defined territory. This is supposed to distinguish the modern state from other, pre-modern forms of control and authority over territories. In pre-modern Europe, in contrast to China, the state did not directly reach every place in a given country. Weber argues that 'the territory must at any time be in some way determinable, but it need not be constant or definitely limited' (Weber, 1978: 901).

Fifth, sovereignty. In addition to the monopolization of violence and effective control over a well-defined territory, sovereignty implies recognition by other sovereign states. The Treaty of Westphalia is generally seen as the point where such a system was initiated to periodically end wars and redraw borders. As wars of aggression were declared illegal by the League of Nations, and then the United Nations, sovereignty in the sense of recognition became an increasingly important tool of survival, primarily for small, resource-poor countries created in the aftermath of decolonization (Jackson, 1990).

Sixth, citizenship. Citizens have a say in the way modern states are constituted and run. Citizenship is expressed through participation in public affairs, and usually regulated by a constitution. This participation is the cornerstone of citizenship, although it may be expressed in various, more or less sophisticated ways.

Seventh, impersonality of authority. One of the key concepts that distinguish modern states from pre-modern ones is the impersonality of power, generally embodied in the rule of law and the bureaucratic system. In modern states, laws apply equally to all citizens and the bureaucracy is expected to ensure they do, without discrimination. But it was also argued that a significant number of modern states have in past decades distanced themselves from the strict, rule-bound, hierarchical and impersonal aspects of public administration (Peters, 1996).

Empirical states may deviate from the above ideal-type features in various ways. Continuity is a key issue. States are created and states may be destructed. States may be divided, or absorbed by larger, more powerful states. Until the nineteenth century, fewer states survived at the end of each war in Europe (Tilly, 1985). In contrast, the dominant trend worldwide in the twentieth century was fragmentation. The number of independent states rose from less than 50 to around 200. A more recent phenomenon is the case of states that, even in the absence of foreign invasion, fade away or even dissolve. In some cases strongmen or warlords constitute a power structure that bypasses the state (Reno, 1998). Weak states sometimes hardly control any territory beyond the capital. The ultimate example is Somalia, which ceased to function as a state in

1991. As a result of these trends, most states have either had a short existence or experienced long periods of discontinuity.

Even the most intrusive states fail to exercise a full monopoly of the legitimate use of force, as violence in prisons illustrates. Weak states may find arrangements with warlords or face open challenges that lead to violent confrontations. States sometimes manage to control such challenges through legislation of exception, but open internal conflicts often spill across borders. In situations of civil war, a shift from the control of territories to the control of populations by warring parties was noted (Jean, 1996; Reno, 1998).

Citizenship is a key issue. Residents of a given territory may be denied citizenship or discriminated against on racial, religious or ethnic grounds. In contrast, non-residents may be granted citizenship on the basis of shared ethnicity, race, religion or other factors.

Sovereignty and territorial control do not always coincide. Some states lack international recognition despite territorial control. Others are recognized even though they hardly control any territory. The Sovereign Order of Malta is an extreme case and enjoys diplomatic ties with 100 countries, even though it has not controlled any territory since 1798 (Sovereign Order of Malta, 2008).

Recognition vs. isolation

In the international system, isolation was sometimes self-imposed, but more often externally imposed. As Western powers dominated the UN until the 1960s, communist states in divided countries (North Korea, East Germany) were kept outside of the organization. In particular, the Republic of China was recognized as the legitimate representative of China, and the People's Republic excluded. The tide turned gradually in the 1950s and 1960s, as a group of anti-communist nations, including South Africa, Chile, Israel, Taiwan and South Korea, faced growing opposition and isolation in the international arena. Although these states became isolated at various dates and on various grounds, they all faced antagonism from the rapidly increasing number of newly independent nations in Africa and Asia in the 1960s and 1970s, aligned with communist and oil-producing countries (Inbar, 1985). Sometimes only the regime was targeted, as in the case of apartheid and Pinochet's Chile, and sometimes the existence of the state itself was threatened, as in the case of Taiwan (Geldenhuys, 1990).

The tide turned again at the end of the Cold War. It was predicted all states would eventually converge towards democracy and market values (Fukuyama, 1992). States that deviated from the new norm were regarded as dysfunctional and ineffective. It was argued that excessive emphasis had been put on formal sovereignty (Jackson, 1990). Quasi-states were unable to effectively control populations on their defined territory, let alone provide basic services to these populations, and sometimes brought trouble to the neighbourhood.

What are the implications for the ways in which states operate as they seek to acquire some form or degree of recognition? Various categories of states can be identified if we combine the two norms of sovereignty and legitimacy, around which the international order is seemingly articulated. Possible categories include liberal democracies, illiberal democracies, undemocratic or unrepresentative regimes, 'rogue' states, ineffective states, and states that have disappeared.

There is no direct correlation between a state's legitimacy and its sovereignty. Some states score highly on both counts and others fail on both counts. Some states or regimes may enjoy high sovereignty and low legitimacy in terms of human rights, such as China, while others have limited sovereignty and high legitimacy, such as Taiwan. In addition, some entities enjoy both high legitimacy and sovereignty in the international order even though they lack a territorial dimension (Vatican, Sovereign Order of Malta).

While all states invoke norms, use organizations and manipulate processes to achieve specific outcomes, states which score low on a given norm may argue it is of little importance. North Korea invokes formal sovereignty and derides the legitimacy that derives from the respect of human rights. In contrast, Taiwan focuses on legitimacy and plays down the recognition aspect of sovereignty.

States with limited recognition may enrol non-state organizations to establish channels of communication with other states. They may even disguise state organizations as formally non-state ones. Conversely, regular states may prefer to use non-state channels to avoid dealing directly or officially with such states.

As norms get twisted and the identity of actors becomes uncertain, interactions between state, market and civil society in the global arena may be characterized by a low degree of transparency when they involve such states. How do we ascertain the identity, mandates and objectives of the actors involved in such cases? To whom are they accountable? What outcomes are they likely to pursue in the global context?

Isolated states may seek increased military power and substantive alliances or other security guarantees, such as formal non-aggression pledges (North Korea with the US, Taiwan with China). Asserting a territorial dimension, such as control over a defined territory or claims over disputed territories, may be even more important for states with low recognition and/or legitimacy than for others. Territorial claims are often linked to control over populations, but may focus on resource-rich territories (like the Spratly Islands).

Control over material resources, including mines, oilfields, pipelines, trading infrastructure, investment and aid, may similarly be even more crucial for unrecognized rulers such as warlords (Tilly, 1985; Reno, 1998). Resource-poor and isolated states may try to extract such resources either by physical threats or by portraying themselves or their citizens as victims. Conversely, a relatively wealthy but isolated state like Taiwan may leverage material resources and use them to acquire physical or symbolic resources.

States seeking to improve recognition may focus on expanding ties with 'regular' states and try to boost their standing through increased interaction with multilateral organizations. Success is difficult to predict, as the shape of the international order is changing. Possible outcomes for states or aspiring states include disintegration, partition, reunification, integration or recognition as a full-fledged, regular state.

Whether legitimate or not, whether recognized or not, states must increasingly deal with a global arena that is organized around specific rules, includes numerous non-state actors and involves them in processes that cut across borders. To help make sense of both domestic and global systems of governance to which states have to respond, the ideas and key elements of governance need to be addressed. The relevance of these ideas and elements can then be explored in the global context in general, and thereafter more specifically in the field of public health and humanitarian action.

Governance discourse and systems

Governance as a set of ideas

Over the past two decades, governance has emerged as a set of ideas that help to describe, analyse and possibly explain the bases and patterns of interaction involving the state, market and civil society. State, market and civil society are used here to describe three distinct, though closely interrelated spheres of human activity. Very broadly, the state primarily has a political base and orientation, the market an economic one, and civil society a social one. Each of these spheres has its own legitimacy and relative autonomy, although the state remains the central actor in governance and is the overriding source of legitimacy (Pierre and Peters, 2005). The legitimacy of the market and civil society is not yet as firmly established in terms of the contributions of their actors to public policy-making and implementation.

Beyond the diversity of ideological approaches and national styles (Peters, 1996; Pierre and Peters, 2005), governance rests on the important underlying idea that a balance should be struck between the different spheres. Overemphasis on one sphere at the expense of others may lead to systemic problems and, in extreme cases, to collapse. In a totalitarian regime, the political sphere absorbs the other two. Alternatively, a weak state may be overwhelmed by economic or social forces it cannot control. These matters are addressed in more detail below.

None of the three spheres is a centralized, unitary entity. This is obviously the case for the market which is driven by competition, and civil society which is marked by pluralism. The state itself has three branches – executive, legislative and judiciary – with each having its own institutions, processes and practices.

Organizations are an important focus of governance, as they are the main institutional mechanisms in or through which actors are aligned and interact within and across the three spheres. Each sphere essentially has an ideal-type organization, but in reality the organizations are of various forms, with numerous public–private overlaps and mixes.

A significant view is that governance is primarily about steering, and can be defined as ‘the process through which public and private actions and resources are coordinated and given a common direction and meaning’ (Pierre and Peters, 2005: 83). In this conception the monopoly of the state over policy-making and policy implementation is challenged, following earlier criticism of the welfare state paradigm and extensive role of the state in the economy (Hayek, 1944; Nozick, 1974).

Governance embraces the idea that the market and civil society can be enrolled along with the state in the provision of these goods. As a result, 'the governance perspective draws on broad strategies of resource mobilization across the public-private border' (Peters and Pierre, 2003: 3). This idea is both empirical and normative. In particular, enrolling a mixture of state and non-state organizations, both for-profit and non-profit, in the delivery of public services may help achieve not only greater efficiency and effectiveness but also greater legitimacy (Peters, 2002a). But it was also argued that while the market model offers an alternative perspective on service delivery, it fails to address other key issues, such as policy advice (Peters, 1996). In addition, as more state and non-state organizations get involved in governance arrangements, the need arises for increased coordination between the various actors and networks, which is frequently a role only the state can fulfil (Thynne, 2000).

The market is the primary arena of economic activities, although the state and civil society also play a role in the economy. Markets are decentralized and ideally based on the respect of such norms as fair competition, openness, efficiency and security (Balaam and Veseth, 2001).

The idea of civil society is more complex and controversial. It is primarily a negative one: civil society is neither market nor state, although it shares some characteristics of both. Like the state, it focuses on collective causes, issues or services. Like the market, it is decentralized and open to competitive efforts.

Key elements of governance

Governance involving the state, market and civil society has a number of interrelated elements. In essence:

- Actors compete for influence over norm-setting, values and principles (Drahos and Braithwaite, 2001; Beier, 2002).
- The emergence of new norms, values and principles may lead to the creation and involvement of new actors.
- Norms, values and principles strongly influence actors and the processes they set in motion.
- Actors obviously influence, and are selective in, the processes utilized.
- The activities of actors in and through various processes result in outputs and outcomes.

More specifically, governance can be seen as an evolving set or system of norms, values and principles which are obviously rooted in a particular historical situation. The governance approach follows the perceived failure of the welfare state, and goes beyond the market-focused privatization drive of the 1980s. This leads to several questions. Is the governance approach the only rational choice in a globalizing world? Or is it just an effective way for developed countries to control and steer the changes globalization induces? How are the underlying norms produced? Do they rest on widely shared values, or on compromises between conflicting values and principles?

The actors include both state and non-state organizations and the people involved. What are their respective mandates, powers, autonomy, goals and resources? How can we categorize organizations? Is it necessary to identify who initiates and controls a given organization, whatever its form? Should organizations themselves be analysed as tools of governance?

The actors adopt processes involving linking arrangements and policy tools. Are processes inclusive of all potential stakeholders, or are they usually exclusive or selective? Are they driven by the quest for consensus? What is the role of the various organizations involved? How much autonomy do they retain or relinquish in the process? What are the bases on which particular policy tools are selected? How does the distribution of power between the various actors affect these processes? What mix of policy tools best suits the governance approach? How effective are these tools?

Actors, influenced by norms and values and adopting specific processes, seek to achieve outputs and outcomes. What are outputs and outcomes, and how might they be distinguished? By what standards or criteria can or should they be evaluated? Should the main focus be on the effective delivery of specific goods and services? Or should it be on desirable outcomes?

Norms, values and principles

Norms are broadly defined here as expected modes of behaviour. Human rights have become a political norm since the 1970s. Whereas scant attention was paid to human rights by states until then, they gradually became a global benchmark in the aftermath of the Helsinki Agreement (1975). Norms evolve in response to changed situations and perceptions. Whereas certain behaviours are expected, the underlying expectations can be changed.

How are norms created? Who defines them? Do these norms rest on a set of widely shared values? Are they the result of a selection process between various views and a wide array of possibilities in a pluralistic arena? Or are they the outcome of clashes or compromises between antagonistic and conflicting values? The acceptance of human rights as a norm may be the result of a wide-ranging, multi-level debate, which has led to a certain consensus. But this may not be the case for a number of other norms. Specific norms are regarded as prerequisites for the governance approach to succeed. In particular, the actors involved are expected to be open-minded and flexible. Governance processes are expected to be open, fair and inclusive. But how inclusive? Does everyone need to be involved, or just a critical mass of actors?

Even if the definition of a given norm is endorsed by actors from all spheres, the distribution of power between the actors must not be overlooked. Some actors may be coerced into an agreement. The state, because of its legitimacy and the range of policy instruments at its disposal, may coerce the market and civil society into the definition of a norm. Conversely, excessive coercion may lead some actors to walk out or criticize, thereby lessening the legitimacy of the exercise. Ultimately, the acceptability of norms, and hence their effectiveness, will depend on the answers to all these questions.

Values inform norms, principles and actions but do not necessarily provide definite answers with regard to a particular course of action. For instance, referring to human rights is useful but does not provide a single answer on the best ways to protect both security and civil liberties. Governance refers to democratic values, such as citizens' participation in policy-making and implementation. Governance also refers to utilitarian values, seeking to achieve the greatest good for the greatest number. Governance can be seen as an effort to articulate the inherent tension between democratic and utilitarian values. Different values may inform different spheres. There is no set convergence of political, economic and social values. This leads to a wider question: who defines and spells out these values – the actors in each sphere? Or are they defined by a procedure everyone agrees on?

Principles can be regarded as primarily value-based operational concepts (for instance, legitimacy, universality, impartiality, neutrality, sovereignty). Flexibility, open-mindedness and inclusiveness have been described as norms, but they can also be seen as stated principles of governance. While norms articulate principles, principles have a stronger grounding in ideas and appear to be less transient than norms. Some of the principles mentioned above, including sovereignty, neutrality or impartiality, have been tried and tested over centuries. They may therefore command a more lasting respect than norms if these norms can be manipulated by powerful actors for their own convenience.

Organizational actors

Governance recognizes that the state, market and civil society each comprise numerous actors which usually operate within or through an array of organizations. Thus, what is an organization? Is it expected to be self-governing and institutionalized in a particular way? Does it have to be formalized and publicized? These are important questions of particular relevance to the organizations addressed in this study.

There are reasons why market or civil society organizations may not register, including the absence of a relevant legal status, the existence of control issues, as traditional forms of governance may be threatened by the requirements of registered organizations, or the intent to carry out illegal or criminal activities. In addition, civil society organizations willing to register may be barred or discouraged from doing so. In particular, authoritarian or colonial governments may prefer not to see their weak legitimacy challenged by legalizing potentially threatening organizations (Sinn, 1989).

There are also various incentives for organizations to register with the relevant authorities, including the threat of penalties for failure to register adequately, the protection against potential liabilities for directors or trustees, and the possibility to raise funds publicly or get access to government contracts and grants. In addition, civil society and non-profit organizations may want to register to offer tax incentives to donors or bring increased recognition to members and volunteers.

There are also reasons why even registered organizations may not want to formalize or publicize all their arrangements. In particular, the activities of non-permanent workers or non-paid volunteers are often less formalized than those of paid staff, which allows added operational flexibility. Arrangements may be kept informal for security reasons (for instance, human rights organizations working in sensitive contexts). Private fundraising can be an attractive option, even for organizations that have the capacity to raise funds publicly. Also, donors or investors may, for various reasons, want to remain anonymous. They may not want to be publicly associated with a controversial cause, charity or company. They may be concerned with privacy protection. Investors may not want to disclose their assets. Donors may choose to remain anonymous for cultural reasons.

Other issues also affect the way organizations can be classified or viewed. Increasingly, the borders between public and private organizations are not clearly delineated. Whereas states are in charge of public affairs, this is also the case with many civil society organizations. There is often a degree of blending in several respects. States may create private organizations with public powers. Or non-state organizations set up under private law may be recognized as public entities (for instance, the International Committee of the Red Cross). What matters primarily is not the private form of these organizations, but their focus on public issues: policy advocacy and/or the delivery of public goods or services (Morris, 2000).

The pursuit of profit is arguably the most important criterion that helps distinguish a market organization from a civil society organization. Is a profit-making organization automatically disqualified as a civil society organization? In most jurisdictions there is nothing that prevents a civil society organization from making a profit. What is prohibited is the distribution of these profits to members or directors. Such 'profit' is simply treated as surplus income and carried forward. Besides, public goods can be delivered by organizations that bring individual benefits to their members (Morris, 2000), such as mutual aid societies and cooperatives. In contrast, trade and industry associations may be formally non-profit but seek benefits for their for-profit members. Do they qualify as civil society organizations? Company foundations are another grey area.

Processes

There is a great diversity of arrangements linking state and non-state actors (Peters, 1988). Of particular interest here are links in which organizations retain their own identity and do not formally merge, but interact in some way. Such horizontal arrangements are variously described as networks, movements, coalitions, coordinations or collaborations (Brown and Keast, 2003). A categorization of 'inter-organisational innovations' (Mandell and Steelman, 2003) distinguishes between intermittent coordination, a temporary task force, permanent and/or regular coordination, a coalition, and a network structure. The authors assess these five steps along six functional characteristics: problem orientation; commitment to goals; intensity of linkages; breadth of effort; complexity of purposes; and scope of effort. Such categorizations help narrow down the huge diversity and variety of arrangements to a manageable level. They also raise the following questions:

Is there a correlation between the duration and the perspective or goals sought by the initiators? A narrow focus or a limited goal may require long-term collaboration. In contrast, a linking arrangement may be set up to pursue system changes in the short term.

Does the degree of formality or the intensity of linkages necessarily increase over time? Long-term efforts may require only intermittent coordination, or loose linkages at certain times and tight linkages at others.

How can inclusiveness be fostered? It has been argued that 'member perceptions and trust influence who is included in the formation and continuation of the arrangement' (Mandell and Steelman, 2003). But it can be argued that organizations which trust each other initially may come to distrust each other after establishing closer links. Conversely, organizations that distrust each other initially may alter perceptions in a process of collaboration and increase mutual trust. In addition, arrangements may link organizations for reasons other than trust (such as interest) or even despite mutual distrust. In particular, it was found that 'the motivations to partner tend to be driven by a desire to secure resources that are more scarce for the respective sector' (Gazley and Brudney, 2007: 411).

How horizontal are such arrangements? There is no symmetry between the various participants, as the government is obviously and legitimately in the driver's seat (Head and Ryan, 2003). As a result, the cost of staying out may be prohibitive for non-state actors, considering the panoply of policy tools at the disposal of the state.

Are all actors equally committed to the purpose of the arrangement? One subgroup of actors, for example the initiators of an arrangement, or those most likely to benefit from the outcomes, may be more committed than another. Alternatively, commitment to goals may depend on the types of actors involved. This echoes earlier remarks on values. A private company must primarily look at its bottom line, as it will disappear if it does not make a profit, however committed to a higher goal its members, management or staff may be. A state organization with multiple mandates cannot commit to just one of these. In contrast, a civil society organization may commit itself to an overriding goal. Indeed, a civil society initiative may not even worry about becoming an organization, as was the case for the International Campaign to Ban Landmines, until it was awarded the Nobel Peace Prize. The issue is complicated when actors make problematic claims. Questioning such claims helps clarify the roles of actors, as was done for corporate social responsibility (Vogel, 2005).

Issues of duration, scope, trust, commitment and inclusiveness are important aspects of linking arrangements. Patterns of interaction between participants also depend, among other things, on the policy tools adopted by the organizations involved.

Policy tools or instruments of public action have increasingly been the focus of public policy studies in the past decades, as frustration increased over the shortcomings of direct delivery of services by governments and third-party actors became involved in the delivery of such services. Salamon (2002) defines a tool of public action as 'an identifiable method through which collective action is structured to address a public problem'.

To help make sense of these tools, it is necessary to limit the number of categories. In particular, Brigham and Brown (1980) categorize tools as either affirmative (encouraging or promoting certain actions or behaviours) or negative (restraining or punishing specific actions or behaviours). Etzioni differentiates between three types of tools: physical (coercive), material (remunerative/utilitarian) and symbolic (normative/persuasive) (Etzioni, 1975). Questioning whether disincentives are covered by Etzioni's classification, Vedung suggests policy instruments can be categorized as sticks (regulations), carrots (economic means) or sermons (information) (Vedung, 1998).

Vedung defines regulation as mandatory, authoritative. However, citizens may choose to disregard the mandatory nature of the law. Regulatory power then requires the additional dimension of physical constraint. It is suggested here that Etzioni's threefold classification of power can be blended with Vedung's emphasis on the negative/affirmative dimension of each category of tools (see Table 2.1).

Physical instruments may either constrain or enable. A government can deliver a passport and enable its holder to travel overseas, or deny it. A government may ban a demonstration, or authorize it. Speed bumps may not discourage all drivers from speeding, but those who do may get hurt. Restrictions to freedom of movement are physical instruments.

Material instruments include costs and benefits, both monetary and in kind. A government may offer cash grants, tax breaks or free services to encourage certain actions or behaviours. In contrast, it can levy taxes on tobacco smokers, fine hunters of endangered species or withdraw food stamps from welfare recipients.

Symbolic instruments are by nature neither physical nor material. Awards and medals are given to outstanding citizens, while slanderers are sentenced to symbolic damages and their condemnations published in the press.

Table 2.1 Policy instruments: a proposed three-way categorization

	Physical	*Material*	*Symbolic*
Negative	Constrain/restrict	Reward/gratify	Shame/warn
Affirmative	Enable/facilitate	Charge/extract	Praise/encourage

Source: adapted from Etzioni (1975) and Vedung (1998).

Policy instruments may be combinations of various elements belonging to different categories. For example, a reckless driver may be shamed by a judicial process (symbolic) and sentenced to jail (physical), but offered a bailout option (material).

Information is not a tool in itself, although it may be useful to enhance the effectiveness of a given instrument. It is probably most essential at the symbolic level (what would be the meaning of secret shaming or praising?) and less so for the physical category (do you have to be reminded that if you murder someone you will go to jail?).

The use of policy instruments may be more or less direct and intense. More importantly, tool selection is not a politically neutral operation and it is not possible to reduce 'instrument selection to the technical exercise of selecting the instrument that is most appropriate for the nature of the policy problem' (Peters, 2002b: 552). In addition, policy instruments are not equally available to all governments. Also, tools are often used in combination or following a particular sequence. Democratic governments tend to use least coercive tools first (Vedung, 1998).

Outputs and outcomes

Outputs consist of concrete and measurable results, such as the total amount of cheques mailed to welfare recipients, the number of policemen recruited, or the total length of highways built within a year. A key issue is whether outputs have positive, acceptable outcomes. For example, increasing welfare payments may be found to be counterproductive, if it encourages recipients to stay out of the workforce. Recruiting more policemen does not necessarily lead to improved security. Similarly, more highways do not necessarily mean fewer traffic jams or accidents. What ultimately is the primary target: more efficiently delivered outputs, or more desirable outcomes?

The answer depends in part on the norms, values and principles of the actors involved. Egalitarian and universal values are more likely to translate into free basic healthcare for all, while utilitarian ones are more likely to result in differentiated levels of service and fees. Ultimately, voters legitimate the policies implemented to achieve targeted outputs or outcomes.

Outputs and outcomes also depend on the expectations of the actors involved and their constituents. Specific interest groups may have very diverse expectations on proposed policy changes. Public policy-making requires articulating and integrating diverse and sometimes conflicting expectations. It is therefore important to make sense of bargaining processes. In addition, 'examination of policy instruments also reveals a great deal about the choices that governments make when they set policy', even though 'the capacity of instrument choices to ensure certain types of outcomes is sometimes overstated by the advocates of one or another instrument' (Peters and van Nispen, 1998: 1–2). Besides, as processes are relatively open, outputs and outcomes may be as unintended as they are unpredictable (Head and Ryan, 2003).

Governance in the global context

The various elements of governance are increasingly significant and complex in the global arena. Governance in the form of global interactions between states, markets and civil societies has increasingly been recognized as important (Rosenau, 1992; Keohane and Nye, 1971; Nye and Donahue, 2000; Weiss and Gordenker, 1996). The global dimension is immediately relevant to this study. States struggle to retain a monopoly on cross-border relations, as an increasing number of non-state actors interact across borders. Norm creation is no longer the monopoly of states. States may find it more difficult to drive processes and achieve targeted outputs and outcomes.

Norms, values and principles

How are norms created in the global context? Should the focus be on legal aspects, such as respect for international law and multilateral agreements, or on the distribution of power between the actors involved?

Norms are often informed by values, rooted in a particular cultural and historical context. Is there a set of values acceptable to all human beings? Is there a process or procedure by which these values can be identified? How do we reconcile the democratic values on which governance is based with the anarchy of the international system? In particular, it was argued that there are competing attempts to define the norms and principles of global governance (Drahos and Braithwaite, 2001).

Organizational actors

Questions of definition and classification also apply to organizations as key elements of governance in general and globally. It is sometimes difficult to distinguish between state, market and civil society organizations. This difficulty may be compounded when we try to make sense of such distinctions across countries. Besides, it may be difficult to categorize some transnational organizations, such as the Catholic Church or the Red Cross.

In the global context numerous actors have to be reckoned with. Intergovernmental organizations (IGOs) may be regional or have a global reach. Such organizations may have overlapping and sometimes conflicting mandates, but eventually all derive their authority from states. Multinational corporations (MNCs) are regarded as the most influential organizations in the market sector. Civil society organizations are less integrated at the global level. However, this may be compensated by their networking capacity, an issue which is returned to below.

In the global context, the legitimacy of organizations in all three spheres may be challenged. In particular, state organizations entrusted with a monopoly over certain functions in a national context, may find this monopoly and also their legitimacy contested by intergovernmental bodies. Market organizations may find the legitimacy they enjoy in a national context contested at a global level. For example, farmers' lobbies may enjoy a high degree of legitimacy in developed countries and face criticism elsewhere, as the subsidies they receive adversely impact the livelihood of farmers in developing countries. Similarly, civil society organizations based in developed countries are sometimes criticized for their lack of sensitivity to survival and livelihood issues in resource-poor countries.

The distribution of power between the various actors is more complex in the global arena. This issue has long been recognized in interstate relations (Waltz, 1979), but is also relevant to the corporate sector. For instance, small or medium-sized firms based in developing countries are unable to compete with transnational corporations (TNCs) in terms of norm-setting, such as the intellectual property regime. Similarly, it has been argued that NGOs based in developed countries drive the global civil society agenda, occupy strategic positions in the UN system, and establish 'internal hierarchies of voice and access within transnational civil society' (Batliwala, 2002: 393).

Processes

Some authors argue that globalization erodes and challenges traditional command styles (Scholte, 2000), while others point to the reduced capacity of any state to control cross-border processes or outcomes, or both (Badie, 2002). Others again show that globalization reinforces the relative power of the most powerful states (Colonomos, 2001).

While realists posit that interactions between states are the only ones that matter (Waltz, 1979), others emphasize that globalization is primarily driven by market forces. Multinational corporations have long recognized the benefits of expanding trade and investment links across borders. Some argue that coalitions of multinational corporations are the main drivers of the agenda for globalization and point to the increasing number of global norms MNCs have established with very little input from either states or civil society.

The emergence of global civil society is emphasized by some scholars (Keck and Sikkink, 1998; Batliwala, 2002; Florini, 2000; Cohen and Rai, 2000). In contrast, others point to a normative vacuum (Taylor, 2002) or lament that 'GCS [Global Civil Society] is made to explain too much on too weak a foundation' (Munck, 2002: 352).

Some authors welcome the global civil society dynamic (Keck and Sikkink, 1998; Florini, 2000), while others are critical (Waterman, 1999; Batliwala, 2002). Others again argue that the increasing complexity of the global system should lead international NGOs to account to multiple stakeholders (Brown and Moore, 2001; Edwards and Hulme, 1996).

Nevertheless, all these authors agree that cross-border linkages between civil society organizations have increased significantly. In particular, Khagram *et al.* (2002) identified three degrees of integration between civil society organizations at a global level: from networks to coalitions, and from coalitions to transnational social movements.

While some scholars focus on cross-border linkages between organizational actors of the same type, others emphasize the emergence of a global public space, where various types of actors compete for global influence (Badie, 2002; Colonomos, 2001). In this conception, the global public space is no longer the monopoly of any category of actors, but a space contested between various types of actors. How do we make sense of the processes at play? Can we identify patterns of collaboration, networking or other linking arrangements? Global public–private partnerships (GPPPs) have been identified in the health sector (Buse and Walt, 2000). Such partnerships are usually initiated and controlled by the corporate sector. NGOs are typically minor partners, even though their role may be important in service delivery. Transnational advocacy networks (TANs) may include NGOs and social movements, parts of IGOs, and branches of national governments (Keck and Sikkink, 1998). Non-state actors may try to enrol unenthusiastic states in their struggle, as shown in the example of the World Jewish Congress versus Swiss banks holding the assets of victims of Nazism (Colonomos, 2001).

Why would organizational actors of different types, with potentially conflicting values, mandates and priorities join forces in the global arena? Do the various actors involved trust each other or share values? Or do they have common objectives or overlapping missions and mandates? If actors of various types share values, at least in part, value-based networks or coalitions may emerge. But heterogeneous coalitions may just be created on the basis of shared objectives and interests. It has been noted that 'Global governance is not simply an uncontrolled, open-ended process, but patterned by institutions and norms that support certain social forces and exclude others' (Franceschet, 2002: 29). As noted by Drahos and Braithwaite (2001), 'theories that concentrate on a single actor, such as realist international relations theory, or a single mechanism, such as rationality, end up giving a poor account of the patterns of regulatory globalisation' (Drahos and Braithwaite, 2001: 123). Although the distribution of power is critical, weak non-state actors can influence the global regulatory agenda, as in the case of the anti-slavery movement.

Also relevant are the resources and tools used in heterogeneous coalitions, as actors of various types may pool resources and combine tools. Although actors of all types may use all kinds of tools, states disproportionately enjoy the use of physical and regulatory power. Market organizations primarily rely on the use of material tools, while civil society initiatives focus on symbolic tools. If tools are more effectively used in combination, this could help explain why organizations of different types coalesce in the global public space.

Outputs and outcomes

Different types of coalitions may focus on different outputs and outcomes. GPPPs are more likely to focus on the delivery of global public goods (GPGs), while transnational advocacy networks may prioritize norm elaboration and norm change.

As the norms that apply in a given country or cultural environment may antagonize values and norms elsewhere, the issue is: what outputs and outcomes are desirable? The ultimate referees in a national setting are voters. But there is no voting procedure at an international level. Outputs and/or outcomes found desirable by voters in a given country may be found inappropriate by voters in another. In particular, actors from developed, industrialized countries, be they state, market or civil society organizations, may have a significantly stronger influence in the definition of global norms, processes, outputs and outcomes than their counterparts in developing countries.

Governance in the context of humanitarian action

The questions and issues raised by governance are especially complex in the global arena. Although the diverse sectors of activity and concern, ranging from security to finance, trade, environment and many others, partly overlap and intersect in many ways, the norms, actors, processes, outputs and outcomes involved may be very different from one sector to the other.

These aspects of governance are very relevant as humanitarian action involves diverse patterns of interaction between or among state, market and civil society organizations both domestically and globally. This multidimensional area of organized activity has some special features in terms of key norms, values and principles, organizational actors involved, processes adopted, and ultimately outputs and outcomes delivered.

The features are inevitably influenced by the nature of humanitarian action itself, which involves responses or sets of responses to emergencies and life-threatening crises. Some of these crises, in particular natural disasters, may be solved in a domestic framework, depending on the scale of the disaster and the resources available in the country. Others, such as conflicts, population displacements, famines or epidemic outbreaks most frequently call for an international response.

Norms, values and principles

Humanitarian law was created in response to historical developments. In the aftermath of the French Revolution, soldiers recruited for the defence of the nation became an expendable resource. A Swiss philanthropist, Henry Dunant, was an eyewitness at the battle of Solferino in 1859, where thousands of wounded soldiers were left dying on the battlefield. He identified the need for internationally accepted norms to take care of wounded soldiers and civilian victims of conflicts, and set out to create a private, independent organization recognized by all states and belligerents to carry out the required relief activities. This led on the one hand to the Geneva Conventions and on the other hand to the creation of the Red Cross movement.

The Geneva Conventions spell out internationally accepted norms with regard to the protection of, and assistance to, non-combatants (i.e. civilian populations and wounded soldiers), and the responsibilities that fall on the warring parties. In particular, when a country is conquered, the occupying powers must provide the population of the occupied territory with adequate food, medical supplies and other basic necessities.

Another stream of international humanitarian law, known as the laws of war or The Hague Conventions, prohibits certain methods and means of warfare.

> Methods of warfare are the tactics or strategy used in hostility against an enemy, in times of conflict. Means of warfare are the weapons or weapons systems used. The only legitimate objective of war is to weaken and overpower the opponent's military forces.
>
> (Bouchet-Saulnier, 2002: 239)

International humanitarian law is thus defined as the sum of these two branches. In recent years, a partial blending of the two streams has occurred, in particular with the development of a treaty to ban the production, use, trade and stockpiling of landmines. Proponents of the treaty argue that landmines should be banned because they indiscriminately target large numbers of innocent civilians and inflict tremendous suffering long after a conflict is over.

In addition to international humanitarian law, laws applicable to situations of conflicts include 'refugee law; conventions on torture, genocide, the rights of the child and human rights; international criminal law; as well as the rules governing peacekeeping and the interstate solidarity mechanism organised within the UN' (Bouchet-Saulnier, 2002: 2).

In the 1990s, international humanitarian law was increasingly challenged by another, emerging norm: humanitarian intervention. The concept of *droit d'ingérence* [right of intervention], was introduced (Bettati and Kouchner, 1987; Deng, 1993). The basic tenet is that states or, preferably, the international community should intervene to stop rulers who massively violate human rights. Empirically, its origin can be traced back to Operation Provide Comfort, designed to help civilian victims of Saddam Hussein's repression after the Gulf War.

On what basis should a humanitarian intervention be decided? How massively must human rights be violated in a given country to legitimize an international intervention? These issues have been studied extensively (Ignatieff, 2002; Nederveen Pieterse, 1998; Teson, 1996; Weiss and Minear, 1993). The intervention paradigm challenges key principles of humanitarian law, including independence, neutrality and impartiality. In particular, intervention was described as 'selective indignation' (Schnabel and Thakur, 2000) following NATO's operation in Kosovo. Some authors have attempted to reconceptualize humanitarian principles (Minear and Weiss, 1995; Ramsbotham and Woodhouse, 1996) but disaster response remains marked by conflicting norms: international humanitarian law and humanitarian intervention. Post 9/11 interventions in Afghanistan and Iraq were driven by security concerns but featured 'humanitarian' elements of governance. These interventions 'and their difficult aftermaths, show the overlap between humanitarian and geostrategic interests' (O'Hanlon and Singer, 2004: 77). The tension between competing norms is here to stay. Notwithstanding the polarized debate on humanitarian norms and principles, there is a general consensus around humanitarian values, as they pervade all cultures.

Organizational actors

National governments have the primary responsibility to respond to disasters in the territories under their control. Where needed, assistance from other states may be called upon either bilaterally or through specialized agencies of the United Nations including the UNHCR, UNICEF, WFP and WHO. The role of the UN Security Council is to handle threats to international peace.

Market organizations usually have a limited role as funders or providers of relief items in conflicts and other disasters, although their profile is rising. Private military companies have specialized in providing security services to embattled governments, but these companies often have strong linkages to the defence ministries of the US and other Western powers. Some companies are involved in services such as transport, logistics and reconstruction in conflict or post-conflict situations. The media, primarily TV, play a key role in mobilizing public opinion, thus pressing state and non-state actors to respond to disasters.

Founded in 1863, the International Committee of the Red Cross (ICRC) is the first modern humanitarian organization. Based in Geneva, the ICRC is a private organization but is also recognized by states. National Red Cross and Red Crescent Societies have been set up in most countries to promote humanitarian principles. The Geneva Conventions recognize a right of initiative for other humanitarian (e.g. independent, neutral and impartial) organizations. Humanitarian organizations must be free from political, religious or other affiliations. They cannot discriminate between victims and must provide assistance in proportion to the needs that they have independently assessed. Most humanitarian organizations are small, but some groups have a global outreach (Guilloux, 2008).

Processes

There is no direct link between the various contexts of humanitarian action. These contexts are defined by the concept of crisis, meaning a break in a previous equilibrium, however shaky this equilibrium may have been (Brauman, 1995). This distinguishes in particular humanitarian action from development aid. A crisis warrants a humanitarian response if it threatens the lives of large groups of people in a short timespan. A critical indicator is the daily mortality rate of the affected population. It is widely accepted that if the rate exceeds 1/10,000, an emergency response is needed.

It is up to the government of a country struck by disaster to coordinate responses. Depending on the nature of the disaster, its extent and existing capacities in the country, the government may call for international aid. Governments may also be wary of other governments' interventionist motives. Natural disasters sometimes affect more than one country, but even large-scale disasters do not necessarily lead to calls for international aid (Guilloux, 2008). Most disasters that elicit an international response happen in resource-poor countries. This is in particular when violent conflict results in large-scale population displacements. Epidemic outbreaks sometimes call for an international response.

Rufin (1993) described the challenges humanitarian organizations faced in the post-Cold War environment. As the Cold War receded, humanitarian action moved from the sidelines of conflicts, where it had been confined to the humanitarian sanctuaries constituted by refugee camps, to the frontlines.

International humanitarian organizations such as the ICRC, MSF and Oxfam are often the first external actors to respond to crises but the role of local communities and authorities is overlooked. While the ICRC 'acts primarily with regard to conflict situations ... emergency action in peacetime is the domain of the national societies and the Federation' (Forsythe and Rieffer-Flanagan, 2007). Assistance and protection may be provided by state organizations on a bilateral basis or channelled through the UN system, in coordination with local and national authorities. Receiving states sometimes oppose such interventions, as in Kosovo, or accept them grudgingly, as in East Timor.

The UN is not a centralized, unitary agent in disaster response, as several agencies, including the UNHCR, UNICEF and WFP have specific mandates and recognized capacities. The UN has set up an Office for the Coordination of Humanitarian Assistance (UNOCHA) to improve coordination between its various components. The UNOCHA effectively disseminates information through its website, reliefweb.org, but has never managed to assert itself against powerful operational agencies. The UNHCR is usually the focal point for coordination in situations of conflict and large-scale population displacement, and holds regular meetings with all agencies involved, including NGOs. Criticism has been directed at the lack of coordination among NGOs, as well as between NGOs and UN agencies (Minear and Weiss, 1995; Weiss and Gordenker, 1996). This is a difficult issue as the number of organizations involved has grown rapidly over the past two decades.

Some companies, especially in the mining and oil sectors, are often of necessity active in war zones. Their role sometimes goes beyond the provision of relief items, as they may be reluctantly driven to provide, directly or indirectly, resources to warring parties.

Humanitarian assistance processes are complicated by humanitarian interventions. Some operations are carried out within the UN framework under the Department of Peacekeeping Operations (DPO). Even in such cases, UN Security Council resolutions do not always provide a clear, workable road map (as was the case in former Yugoslavia). Increasingly, though, troops operate either outside the UN command (as did US troops in Somalia), bilaterally by delegation of the UN Security Council (as with the US in Haiti or the French in Rwanda) or through regional mandates (as was the case in Sierra Leone and Liberia with the ECOWAS under Nigerian command). Interventions are sometimes launched without a Security Council mandate, as with NATO in Kosovo.

In addition to military involvement, states may use physical tools such as rescue teams, air transport or other logistical services. In contrast, states may constrain humanitarian agencies – for instance, restrict access to disaster areas on various grounds. Governments may also use material tools, such as grants to affected states and humanitarian organizations, or symbolic tools. They may praise relief efforts selectively or shame warring parties that hamper the assistance process.

Although the co-optation of humanitarian action has become an established foreign policy tool, research on the role of humanitarian organizations in a country's foreign policy has been limited, and primarily focused on the United States (Natsios, 1997; Cuny, 1993). NGOs have sometimes been described as implementing agents of foreign policy objectives, even though this role has not been systematically studied (Natsios, 1996).

At first sight it may seem paradoxical to think of competing transnational coalitions in disaster relief, but it was argued that some Islamic states, including Sudan, supported Islamist NGOs to drive out Western relief agencies and regain control of Muslim civilian populations (Bellion-Jourdan, 1997; Ghandour, 2002).

Outputs and outcomes

In a rescue phase during a crisis, a few lives are saved at a great cost. This is for instance the case when specialized rescue teams are flown in to search for earthquake survivors. Setting up a war surgery operation in a conflict area also requires sizeable resources in terms of skills, maintenance of a complex logistical chain, and funds.

Forced population displacements in resource-poor areas often lead to large numbers of casualties among non-combatants. As the size of humanitarian operations and the number of actors increased, their effectiveness was questioned and lack of focus criticized. NGOs were found useful because they helped people UN agencies could not reach, but patterns of UN sub-contracting to NGOs failed to maximize accountability and efficiency (Duffield, 1997; Smillie, 1997; Smith and Weiss, 1997). Minimum standards, where applied with proper understanding of the political context, help lower the number of casualties significantly. Codes of conduct on issues ranging from drug donations to refugee care were drafted jointly by UN agencies and international NGOs. While enforcement remains voluntary, signatories claim to lead by example. Responses to epidemics may require the timely production of an adequate amount of vaccines by the private sector, effective cold-chain management and technical support.

It is more difficult to measure the output and outcomes of humanitarian action in terms of protection than in terms of assistance. Rwanda, Bosnia and many other crises highlighted severe limitations in the level of protection humanitarian organizations can provide. The low level of security and protection in refugee camps is a pervasive issue.

Humanitarian interventions contributed to blurring the identities and roles of NGOs, UN agencies and the military. The growing importance of humanitarian action, or the appearance of it, at the core of global governance must be emphasized. In the 1990s, humanitarian aid became one of the core tools of conflict regulation. This may have happened by default, due to the cost (both financial and symbolic) of alternatives, including peacekeeping and other forms of direct military involvement. Leading humanitarian organizations denounced the use of so-called 'humanitarian' aid by states as an alibi for political inaction.

Duffield (2001) goes one step further and argues that the aid and intervention system represents the limit of a liberal global governance system that responds to state failure with relief operations and acceptance of limited warfare, under the threat of full-fledged war if needed. Humanitarianism should not be seen as a lack of political action, but as that very action, which includes 'the repackaging of development assistance as structural conflict prevention' (Duffield, 2001: 120).

The role of humanitarian action as a key component of conflict management led to a paradoxical situation for independent aid organizations. While their independence was increasingly challenged, they rose to prominence on the international stage. Stepping out of the rank and file of NGOs accredited with the ECOSOC, a select few were invited to speak, for the first time ever, at a United Nations Security Council meeting on the Great Lakes crisis in 1997. This was seen as reinforcing the hierarchy of access (Alger, 2002). It also highlighted the potential danger of what has been described as a 'Faustian bargain' for NGOs (Peters, 2002a: 169), where increased recognition may lead to co-optation and a loss of autonomy.

Fundamental questions were raised about the missions and mandates of humanitarian NGOs (DeWaal, 1997; Jean, 1996). Donini (1995) established that the input of humanitarian NGOs was significant in shaping the policy response of governments, but suggested that the outcome of their activities in the field was questionable. DeWaal (1997) criticized NGOs for their inadequate political analyses and insufficient understanding of the contexts in which they operate. He rightly pointed to the overextended and frequently conflicting responsibilities and activities carried out by NGOs in disaster areas. Indeed, independent humanitarian organizations argue that compromising independence, neutrality or impartiality increases risks for people in war zones and humanitarian workers.

The most difficult dilemmas were discussed long before the current focus on governance in the global context. Does humanitarian action unintentionally prolong wars, if it unwittingly provides physical, material and/or symbolic resources to warring parties? How can humanitarian organizations assist refugees tightly controlled by militias or other warring parties? This issue came to the fore in 1994–95, when half-a-million Hutu refugees from Rwanda fled to Goma in Eastern Congo (Terry, 2002). Humanitarian agencies were criticized for feeding and providing resources to thousands of people who, a few months earlier, had committed genocide.

Analytical framework: a summary

The analytical framework developed here focuses on the interactions of states and governance. It rests on the idea that not only greater effectiveness, but also greater legitimacy can be achieved if non-state actors, whether for-profit or non-profit, are involved in the formulation and implementation of specific policies, even though the state remains the legitimate driver of the process.

The key elements of the governance framework introduced here are norms and values, actors (people and organizations), processes (linking arrangements between the actors and policy instruments), outputs and outcomes. Actors compete over norm-setting and are influenced by existing norms. Governance processes are primarily informed by the interaction of norms and actors. The focus is here on arrangements through which distinct organizations interact in some way and policy instruments. Lastly, influenced by norms and values, actors seek to achieve outputs and outcomes through specific processes.

There is an added degree of complexity in the global arena, as no single actor enjoys the kind of legitimacy that the state enjoys in a national setting. In particular, an important issue is the legitimacy of global norms. Humanitarian action has its own set of contested norms.

States may respond to global governance systems in various ways, enthusiastically or reluctantly. This study focuses on the interactions of an irregular state, Taiwan, with the global systems that seek to respond to diseases and disasters. In the next chapter, the interactions of state and society in Taiwan are examined in a governance framework. This sets the stage for the two case studies that follow: Taiwan's WHO campaign and Taiwan's medical cooperation and humanitarian assistance to developing countries. The primary focus is on the various dimensions of Taiwan's involvement in the relevant global governance systems and the ways in which Taiwan uses elements of these systems to achieve specific objectives.

3 Taiwan

State, governance and society in perspective

Introduction

This chapter sets the scene for the empirical case studies that follow. Taiwan's state and society are introduced here in historical perspective. State is used here as one of the three types of governance actors and organizations identified in Chapter 2, not as an assessment of the legitimacy of Taiwan's arguments in favour of international recognition. Society refers to the actors and organizations identified in the previous chapter as market and civil society organizations. The characteristics of the state, in many ways unique, are introduced first. The complex and diverse patterns of interaction between state and society in the context of Taiwan are then highlighted. In the last section the focus is on state–civil society interactions in external relations.

An irregular state

A disputed status

Of all states, whether regular, contested or aspiring, Taiwan's situation is unique. This is not just because Taiwan is the most significant of all irregular states in terms of economic development and trading power. Taiwan claims it is a sovereign country and fulfils nearly all standard criteria for statehood. The Republic of China effectively controls a specified territory, which includes not only Taiwan but the islands of Jinmen, Matsu and several others, and the entire population residing in these territories. Taiwan regards as irrelevant Beijing's claim of sovereignty, as the PRC has never exercised effective control over any part of these territories.

In support of its argument, Taiwan also emphasizes the size of its population and economy. With 23 million inhabitants, Taiwan is more populated than nearly three-quarters of UN members. Taiwan therefore argues that its exclusion from the global community, and in particular from the United Nations and its specialized agencies, signifies a grave breach of the principle of universality. Taiwan also emphasizes its economic and financial weight, which featured prominently during its campaign to be admitted as a WTO member. Taiwan ranks seventeenth in terms of GDP and is the fifteenth largest trading entity in the world (*Central News Agency*, 20 July 2005).

China's reply to these arguments is that Taiwan is part of China, and that Resolution 2758 of the United Nations General Assembly of 25 October 1971 settled once and for all the question of the representation of China. Passed by 76 votes for, 35 against and 17 abstentions, this resolution recognized the Peoples' Republic as the sole legitimate representative for the whole of China. Beijing therefore states that the Republic of China has no valid claim to sovereignty and membership of the United Nations.

Taiwan is isolated in terms of official diplomatic recognition. The island was described as 'financially rich but diplomatically poor' (Chan, 1997a: 37). This leads to specific questions related to governance elements in this context, first and foremost regarding the nature of Taiwan. Taiwan closely resembles what was defined in Chapter 2 as a state, but does not fulfil all the requirements. Does this really matter in terms of governance? In particular, does this bear on the norms Taiwan refers to? Are these norms different from the norms other states invoke? Another issue is Taiwan's approach to governance processes. Does its atypical status lead Taiwan to use a different set of policy instruments or use them in ways other states would not? If Taiwan's situation is unique, what are the consequences for the state and non-state organizations involved in governance processes? To answer these questions, it is necessary to highlight briefly the historical steps that have led to Taiwan's unique situation and contested status, before turning to the evolution of the state and the evolution of Taiwanese society.

Taiwan's troubled history

Some states fail to control all the territories they claim are under their sovereignty. Other entities may remain in an institutional limbo for a long time but clearly aspire to statehood. The institutional limbo may therefore be described more aptly as a waiting room. In contrast, there is no consensus on what Taiwan is: a de facto independent state or a remote province destined to be sooner or later reunited with the motherland?

Some argue that the ultimate goal is for both sides to be reunited, as happened with Germany and Vietnam and is expected to eventually happen with Korea. Two theories in particular focus on the prospect of reunification: integration theory and the divided nation model. According to integration theory, the gradual development of links between the two sides, starting with economic cooperation, will ultimately lead to political unification. Economic integration is expected to be a stepping stone in a political unification process designed to remedy a perceived aberration (Kuo, 1995; Deng, 2000). Integration theory takes a leaf from the process of gradual integration in Europe. But the prime motive for European integration was political, i.e. to maintain peace in Europe. Economic integration was designed as a process facilitating and leading to political integration. The basic premise across the Taiwan Strait is missing. There is no consensus in Taiwan on the twin issues of economic and political integration with the mainland. In addition, the PRC has not renounced the military option. There is confusion here between hope and reality.

The same applies to the divided nation model (Cheng, 1995). While Vietnam, Germany and Korea were divided by the Cold War, the division of China was the result of civil war, not external constraint. And the history of the KMT regime moving across the strait to take over a freshly decolonized island sets it apart from these other cases where nations that had clearly shared a common history were divided by the Cold War.

The depth and breadth of Taiwan's historical links with the mainland has been a subject of debate for a long time. In spite of two Chinese military expeditions in the third and sixth centuries, 'no massive settlement began until General Cheng Ch'eng-kung (Koxinga, 1624–62) expelled the Dutch from Taiwan in 1661' (Shaw, 1979: 8). Prior to this operation, 'Taiwan and P'eng-hu had been under the molestation of both foreign traders and adventurers and Chinese pirates' (Shaw, 1979: 8). Taiwan was the target of incursions by the Japanese and colonization by Spain and Holland for various periods in the seventeenth century. In the next two centuries, Taiwan was treated with suspicion by Qing dynasty officials because of its connections with Ming loyalists. Taiwan was frontier land and had to be brought under Qing rule to prevent rebels or foreign powers using the island as a base to attack China's coastal provinces. At the same time, the immigration policy was restrictive as China struggled to control the restive province. The policy was gradually relaxed but not fully liberalized until the Japanese attack on Taiwan in 1874 made it obvious that Taiwan had to be populated and rapidly developed if it were to be defended effectively (Shaw, 1979).

Ceded by China at the treaty of Shimonoseki, Taiwan became a Japanese colony for the next 50 years. In spite of colonial discrimination, the Japanese were credited with important developments in Taiwan. One of them was the establishment of law and order, a feature that according to some was lacking prior to Japanese colonization (Wu, 1995). The island's economy developed, though in a traditional colonial conception, where Taiwan supplied raw materials such as tea and sugar, while the colony was regarded as a market for Japanese manufacturing industries. The Japanese are also credited with developing mass education more effectively than other colonial powers in Asia (Shaw, 1979). In addition, and although few natives could become part of the ruling elite, elections took place at the local level after 1935 (Wu, 1995) but decentralization and local autonomy remained very limited (Mengin, 2007).

On the mainland, the Qing dynasty was overthrown and the Republic of China founded by Sun Yat-sen in 1911. Taiwan was reunited with the mainland in 1945. The international recognition of the Republic of China's sovereignty over Taiwan was acknowledged by Roosevelt and Churchill in the Cairo Declaration of 26 November 1943, which stated in particular that 'all the territories Japan has stolen from the Chinese, such as Manchuria, Formosa, and the Pescadores, shall be returned to the Republic of China' (Cairo Declaration, 1943). The Cairo Declaration was later approved by Stalin, and its terms reiterated in the Potsdam Proclamation of 26 July 1945, also endorsed by France. These terms were accepted by Japan when it surrendered on 2 September 1945.

The ROC took over Taiwan on 25 October 1945 (Chiu, 1979). Two months later China became a founding member of the United Nations and one of the five permanent members of Security Council.

Following the defeat of the Nationalists by the Communists on the mainland, Chang Kai-shek retreated to Taiwan in 1949 with a large part of his army and over one million mainlanders. The ROC was initially written off by the US, as it was expected that the PRC would invade Taiwan, but the US changed its policy when war broke out on the Korean peninsula. In particular, the US managed to keep open the question of Taiwan's international status when a peace treaty was signed with Japan in 1952 (Chiu, 1979). As few countries initially recognized the PRC, the ROC kept representing China in the United Nations and other international organizations for more than two decades.

From 'P5' to international pariah

As a permanent member of the Security Council, the Republic of China's international status was at the time the highest possible in the international order. In addition Taiwan gained importance strategically at the outset of the Korean War as one of the frontlines of the Cold War, and one of the staunchest allies of the United States.

Global political trends started eroding Taiwan's international standing. As more and more countries became independent and were admitted as members of the United Nations, Western countries and their allies gradually lost ground. Although many of the newly-independent countries joined the Non-Aligned Movement, the group tended to vote with the Soviet Bloc at the United Nations General Assembly. Predictably, the number of votes in support of the PRC increased over the years (Wang, 1984). Finally, the rift between the Soviet Union and the PRC led the United States to change its China policy and establish links with the Peoples' Republic.

The ROC was eventually expelled from the United Nations in 1971 or, more accurately, withdrew from the organization just before it was stripped of its status as the legitimate representative of China. The sequence of events helps throw light on Taiwan's current efforts to be readmitted. At the 1970 General Assembly of the United Nations, the number of countries which voted in favour of the PRC as the legitimate representative of China for the first time exceeded those in favour of Taipei (Wang, 1984). Even though the US relied on the 'important question' rule, that required a two-thirds majority in the General Assembly, the ROC's expulsion was only a matter of time. In the early months of 1971, the US sounded the Nationalist government on the possibility of dual representation for China. Although the Nationalists were reluctant to agree to such a formula and argued it would legitimize the Communist regime across the Strait, they felt they had no choice.

In July 1971, US Secretary of State Henry Kissinger left for his first secret visit to Beijing, paving the way for a rapprochement with Beijing. The US, in particular its UN ambassador George Bush, officially kept working towards a formula of dual representation, whereby Taiwan would have kept its seat in the General Assembly and transferred its permanent membership of the Security Council to the PRC. But in talks with Zhou En Lai, Kissinger had already written off Taiwan's UN seat and agreed that the US would not raise the 'important question' rule at the upcoming General Assembly meeting of the United Nations. This paved the way for the Peoples' Republic's entry into the United Nations.

During the General Assembly it became clear that the dual representation formula was unacceptable to Chiang Kai-shek, as this would have meant somehow legitimizing the Communist regime on the mainland. As a result, just before the yearly Albanian resolution in favour of Beijing was tabled, Taiwan's envoy, Liu Chieh, delivered the Republic of China's last statement at the United Nations on 25 October 1971:

> In view of the frenzied and irrational manners that have been exhibited in this hall, the delegation of the Republic of China has now decided not to take part in any further proceedings of this General Assembly ... We shall continue to struggle with like minded Governments for the realisation of the ideals upon which the United Nations was founded and which the General Assembly has now betrayed.
>
> (cited in Garver, 1997: 259)

The ROC's claim to represent a territory it did not control eventually backfired. Although it was clear its diplomatic status would inevitably decline with the admission of new members following decolonization, the degree or intensity of its isolation was also of its own making.

Taiwan was regarded as an isolated/pariah state (Vale, 1997; Geldenhuys, 1990) like Israel, South Africa, Chile, and sometimes South Korea. Paradoxically, its diplomatic isolation became more acute as its economic clout grew. Taiwan's diplomatic isolation increased over time as most countries, which had generally wanted to normalize ties with Beijing but were wary of the US reaction, switched diplomatic recognition to the PRC.

In 1988 Taiwan established a new policy, described as 'flexible' or 'pragmatic', to try and break isolation. Taiwan was no longer opposed to dual recognition, i.e. establishing official diplomatic relations with countries that recognized the PRC. The overall objectives were to strengthen ties with official allies, improve and upgrade ties with other countries, and raise Taiwan's profile in international organizations.

Although the ROC managed to establish diplomatic relations with eight Asian and Caribbean countries between 1989 and 1992, the PRC retaliated and wooed the ROC's last three allies of some influence: Saudi Arabia, South Korea and South Africa (Clough, 1999). In addition, Taiwan's official diplomatic ties were under threat from a full-fledged diplomatic offensive of the PRC. Some countries switched official diplomatic recognition from the PRC to Taiwan, such as São Tomé and Príncipe, and Gambia. Others moved in the other direction, such as Niger and South Africa. Others again, such as Senegal, Liberia and Chad, switched from the PRC to Taiwan, and then back to the ROC within a decade. Flexibility has failed to break diplomatic isolation, as no country maintains official ties with both the PRC and the ROC. Barring the special case of the Vatican, Taiwan's 23 official allies (as of 1 August 2008) have little clout or influence.

Taiwan's drive for global recognition

Although this 'non-exclusive' approach has yet to yield results in terms of official bilateral diplomatic ties, it has helped Taiwan seek admission or readmission to intergovernmental organizations. In particular, Taiwan succeeded in gaining membership of IGOs where the PRC is also a member, notably APEC and the WTO.

Taiwan is currently a member of 13 conventional IGOs (Union of International Associations, 2004). The Republic of China was expelled from most UN specialized agencies in the immediate aftermath of the 1971 General Assembly debacle. A new low was reached in 1980, as Taiwan was expelled from the Bretton-Woods institutions (IMF, World Bank, IFC and IDA), to which the PRC had thus far paid little attention. Since then, Taiwan has gained membership of a few intergovernmental organizations thanks to pragmatic diplomacy. In addition, Taiwan was able to channel aid through regional development banks, including the European Bank for Reconstruction and Development (EBRD), African Development Bank, CABEI and Inter American Development Bank.

In 1986, the Asian Development Bank was the first intergovernmental organization to accept both Taiwan and the PRC as members. APEC followed suit in 1991 and the WTO in 2001. The IGOs that accepted both Taiwan and the PRC as members were described as showing flexibility in terms of membership policies (Chan, 1997b). In particular, these organizations have various categories of membership. Full-fledged membership of intergovernmental organizations is usually limited to states, but in some instances other entities such as local governments or non-state organizations may apply for associate membership or other categories of membership. Taiwan was never allowed to join any international organization as a sovereign country. In particular, Taiwan joined the WTO as a 'customs territory', APEC as an 'economy' and various regional fisheries-management organizations as a 'fishing entity'.

> 'We were admitted to these organizations as a "fishing entity" because the related 1995 United Nations Implementing Agreement created the term "fishing entity" and thus allowed some room for flexibility for Taiwan,' Chiang said. Part of Article One of the 1995 UN document states that the agreement 'applies *mutatis mutandis* to other fishing entities whose vessels fish on the high seas'.
>
> (*Taipei Times*, 13 April 2002)

The issue here is not just the nature of the applicant, but its name. Taiwan was never allowed to apply under the name of 'Taiwan' or 'the Republic of China', but only under the names 'Taipei, China', 'Chinese Taipei' or 'the customs territory of Taiwan, Jinmen and Matsu'. Taiwan even tried to disguise itself as an NGO in order to expand its own diplomatic space. In particular, Taiwan is a member of the Unrepresented Nations and Peoples Organization (UNPO):

> Its members are indigenous peoples, occupied nations, minorities and independent states or territories who have joined together to protect their human and cultural rights, preserve their environments, and to find non-violent solutions to conflicts which affect them. UNPO provides a legitimate and established international forum for member aspirations and assists its members in effective participation at an international level. Although UNPO members have different goals and aspirations, they share one condition – they are not represented in major international fora, such as the United Nations. As a result, their ability to participate in the international community and to have their concerns addressed by the global bodies mandated to protect human rights and address conflict, is limited.
>
> (Unrepresented Nations and Peoples Organization, undated)

Taiwan is obviously an economic giant among the 63 members of the UNPO. In addition, Taiwan recently announced the creation of an 'international non-governmental body grouping its diplomatic allies and representatives from the United States, Japan and Australia in another attempt to ease its diplomatic isolation' (*South China Morning Post*, 2 August 2005). Named the Democratic Pacific Union (DPU), this organization 'will have 11 members from the Americas, six from Asia and seven from the South Pacific' (*South China Morning Post*, 2 August 2005). Then Vice-President Annette Lu Hsiu-lien hoped that the DPU, although set up as an NGO, would evolve into an intergovernmental organization. The key point here is that, although Taiwan insists it is a state, it does not rule out unconventional means to promote its claim and attain the status of a fully recognized state.

Taiwan's status in the IGOs it was allowed to join remains precarious. In particular, when it hosted an APEC meeting in Shanghai, the Peoples' Republic refused to invite Li Yuan-zu, a senior advisor to President Chen Shui-bian, as requested by Taiwan, on the ground that the APEC protocol stipulated that an 'economics leader' should attend (Australia-China Chamber of Commerce and Industry of New South Wales, 2001). In 2003 China 'pressured the WTO secretariat to change Taiwan's title used in the directory from a "permanent mission" to an "office of permanent representative" so the title does not imply sovereignty' (*Taipei Times*, 10 May 2004). China even tried to block Taiwanese journalists from covering events such as the World Health Assembly, which drew criticism from President Chen Shui-bian:

> Everyone knows why Taiwan's journalists cannot obtain press permits to report from the WHA. And everyone knows that press freedom represents the consensus viewpoint of the international community and a universal value, and

> that it is also one of the ideals that the United Nations aspires to. Nevertheless, using the excuse that Taiwan is not a member of the United Nations, China pressures the WHA Secretariat to block press accreditation being issued to Taiwan's journalists. This deprives not only Taiwan's journalists of their press rights but also Taiwan's 23 million people of their right to information.
>
> (Office of the President, Republic of China (Taiwan), 2006)

Maintaining hard-earned though limited diplomatic recognition is therefore a permanent challenge for Taiwan. Taiwan's presence in IGOs remains limited to specialized and relatively obscure organizations, barring APEC, the ADB and the WTO. Taiwan's UN campaign was launched in 1993 as seven of its Central American allies sent a memorandum to the UN Secretary-General (United Nations, 1993). The move was countered by China's representative, who sent a note to the UN describing Taiwan's actions as an attempt to split China and scuttle reunification (Chiu, 1998). Although Taiwan's Central American allies reiterated the move in subsequent years, the General Committee never agreed to include the issue of Taiwan's representation in the agenda of the General Assembly.

Separately, Taiwan started a campaign to be readmitted, as an observer, to the World Health Organization, from which the 'representatives of Chiang Kai-shek' were expelled in 1972 (World Health Organization, 1973: 353). Taiwan's WHO campaign is the focus of one of the case studies (see Chapters 4 and 5).

The survival imperative

Due to its small size and precarious status, Taiwan's options are limited. Taiwan tries to compensate this with US support, advanced technology and tight integration in the global economy. This lends itself well to an effective defensive posture considering the width of the Taiwan Strait, although the constant build-up of military capacities on the mainland makes Taiwan's position critical in the long term. In particular, it was argued that 'Israel continues to exist for two simple reasons: first, because it possesses a first rate military capability and, second, because the United States supports its existence' (Niou, 1995: 205). After discussing Taiwan's options, the author concludes that 'to secure the ROC's survival, both the first and the second policies, enhanced military capability and alliance building with the United States, are self-evident. The value of the third policy – focused on ending Taiwan's diplomatic isolation – is debatable' (Niou, 1995: 209).

Taiwan's survival as a self-governing entity depends on US military support. This support was unequivocal from the beginning of the Korean War in 1950 until the US switched recognition to the PRC in the 1970s. The US has since tried to maintain a balance between the two sides of the Taiwan Strait. On the one hand it recognizes the PRC and follows a one-China policy. On the other hand, the US discourages military adventurism and supports peaceful reunification between the two sides. In particular, when the PRC flexed its muscles in the 1995–96 crisis, following President Lee Teng Hui's visit to America, the US despatched two aircraft carrier battle groups to the strait. It was argued that the US position evolved and tilted towards the PRC when US President Clinton, in remarks made in Beijing and Shanghai, appeared 'to have shifted from comfort with the status quo over Taiwan to supporting a peaceful reunification of the two Chinas' (Chou, 1999: 120). But the US has maintained strategic ambiguity and kept both sides guessing how it would respond to open conflict. It was also argued that

> the record of US policy over Taiwan since the normalization of US–PRC diplomatic relations has witnessed both periods when the US leaned to the PRC side and cut back ties with Taiwan and periods when the US endeavoured to stand firm in support of US interests in Taiwan despite pressures from Beijing.
>
> (Sutter, 1999: 177)

The US has consistently delivered defensive weapons to Taiwan to counter the military build-up undertaken by the PRC. The threat is clear, and Taiwan's vulnerability equally clear. In line with the power asymmetry theory it was argued that the choice for Taiwan is between balancing (increasing defence capabilities) and bandwagoning (falling in line with the PRC) (Wu, 2000). In addition, Taiwan sought to enrol society in efforts to bolster its position. The evolution of the links between state and society is now examined.

State–society interactions

Authoritarian rule, democratization and Taiwan's identity

Taiwan started as an authoritarian state. The imposition of martial law from 1949 onwards was regarded as a necessity and a consequence of the civil war and partition (Mengin, 1999). In accordance with the Constitution of the Republic of China, drafted in 1936 and enacted in 1947,

> the office of president is a powerful one in that he is not only the commander of the armed forces and nominates or appoints key officers for the government, such as the premiership, but is also endowed with the power to make emergency decrees.
>
> (Wang, 1994: 126)

Nonetheless, the view that the KMT was a quasi-Leninist party was challenged and it was argued that, although the KMT borrowed methods and principles from this model, such as democratic centralism, it never became a truly Leninist organization (Tsang, 1999).

Taiwan has been described as a strong developmental state. Developmentalism was used in the Latin American context to characterize states that considered 'economic performance the most important basis upon which a regime may claim legitimacy' (Gong and Chen, 1996: 22). In this conception, the state is the prime mover in the economic sphere and the goal of economic development calls for enhanced administrative capacity (Gong and Chen, 1996). The term was also used in the context of Japan and referred to state-driven modernization, both in terms of capacity and determination. This included the ability to mobilize society and corporations (X. Huang, 2001). But Huang also argued that 'the popular interpretation that an East Asian-type growth tends to be associated with an authoritarian state has gone beyond what was intended by the concept of the developmental state, and has consequently led to confusions and intense debates' (X. Huang, 2001: 139).

More pointedly, the developmental state paradigm focuses on two distinct issues: state autonomy, or authority, and state capacity (X. Huang, 2001; Leng, 1996).

> State capacity is a set of institutional arrangements underlying the effectiveness of the government's policy formulation and implementation, while authority structure is a set of relationships among primary forces in a given social environment that reflect, as well as enforce, a distribution of political power.
>
> (X. Huang, 2001: 141)

Taiwan's new rulers were initially more radically separate from the society they set out to rule than most other Asian or Latin American strong states. The KMT regime was regarded as the ultimate strong state as it had no ties or allegiance to the local elites. One million mainlanders moved to Taiwan in 1949 and took control of the island. The martial law was declared and maintained until 1987. During this period the state was able to impose land reform, silence labour and control business (Leng, 1996).

But Leng argues that 'the strong-state paradigm also has its weaknesses. One salient characteristic is its 'unevenness' over time and in different policy spheres' (Leng, 1996: 10). Another problem is that 'the strong-state paradigm also fails to analyze the political economy of the East Asian newly industrialized countries (NICs) in the era of democratic transition' (Leng, 1996: 10).

Authoritarianism was seen as the necessary entry point for a regime under siege (Mengin, 1999), but the nature of this authoritarianism was also questioned. While coercive measures were used, the importance of ideological campaigns should not be understated (Chu, 2001). The KMT regarded itself as the only legitimate government of China after retreating to Taiwan. Objectives and slogans were thereafter adjusted to take stock of geopolitical evolutions, from 'Develop Taiwan, then recover the Mainland with glory' in the 1950s to 'Construct Taiwan to be the model province of the Three principles of the People' when re-conquering the mainland appeared increasingly unrealistic (Chu, 2001). Ideological measures were systematically backed up by organizational drives.

> Mobilisational authoritarianism was based on the idea that obedience rendered under coercion is a less reliable foundation for a state (especially a state at war, which the ROC considered itself to be until 1991) than voluntary

> cooperation. Both Sun Yat-sen and Chiang K'ai-shek emphasised the importance of enmeshing citizens in public life by involving them in a vanguard party and its subsidiary organisations. The notion that citizens needed to be mobilised behind a revolutionary party was central to Sun's theory of political tutelage and development.
>
> (Rigger, 1996: 301)

The democratic transition in Taiwan was smoother and more gradual than in other East Asian countries. Ku (2002) identified four phases in the process: authoritarianism (1949–72); semi-democracy (1972–88); the transition toward democracy (1988–96); and democratic consolidation thereafter. He also emphasized that 'mass political participation and democratic consolidation do not come overnight' (Ku, 2002: 75) and argued that 'a change in type of regime is not necessarily connected with economic development' (Ku, 2002: 74). While the link between economic development and regime change may not be direct, Wu (1995) contends that 'the ability of the government to initiate effective economic policies has allowed Taiwan to attain a fairly high level of socioeconomic development, which has proved to be very important in pressuring the government to relax its rigid political control' (Wu, 1995: 12).

Legislative elections were not conducted on the island after 1949 on the grounds that the objective of the Republic of China was to recover the mainland, that legislators had been elected nationwide in 1946, and that given the state of war it was not possible to organize such representative elections. But a slow democratization process took place nonetheless.

> Despite the martial-law regime, people in Taiwan began to practice direct elections at the local level in the early 1950s, creating a foundation for Taiwan's later democratization. Taiwanese political participation was expanded to the national level in December 1969, when eleven legislators to the Legislative Yuan and fifteen delegates to the National Assembly were directly elected by the people in the Taiwan area.
>
> (Ku, 2002: 59)

In the decades that followed, an organized opposition gradually emerged. One of the main themes, if not the overriding one, was the expression of a distinct identity. In contrast with the dominant KMT discourse, the opposition claimed that Taiwanese society was distinct from Chinese society due to historical factors and various foreign influences over the past centuries. Democratic aspirations and flexible diplomacy were therefore enmeshed with the identity issue from the start (Kuan, 2006). Internally, Taiwanese became increasingly assertive. Externally, soul-searching led to a quest for international standing. Mengin (2007) showed how Taiwan's democratization was intrinsically linked to the geographical re-definition of the state.

It was argued that the status quo in cross-strait relations could be maintained, as all parties in an open electoral competition try to maximize votes and most

Taiwanese voters want neither independence nor reunification (Wu, 2000). While empirical support was found for the hypothesis that political parties converged in the 1990s, it is unclear whether this has been the case since 2000 (Fell, 2004). Taiwan's democratic credentials are not the issue here. But Taiwan's unclear status sets it apart from other, 'normal' democracies. The hidden assumption behind the vote-maximizing model is that of an unquestionable, shared collective identity. The situation in Taiwan is different. Some voters consider themselves to be primarily Chinese and others Taiwanese, as Taiwan's identity was shaped by colonization and complex patterns of migration (Chang, 2000). Besides, Taiwanese perceptions of identity are not set in stone but fluid and subject to -evolution (Lin, 2001). Where identity was a major issue, electoral politics often radicalized positions and led to violent conflict. In this regard, the peaceful demise of Czechoslovakia may be the exception rather than the rule. Mengin argues that 'at a time when ideologies are passing away, the identity discourse may well replace – and in some cases, such as the former Yugoslavia, have replaced – them' (Mengin, 1999: 126). Mengin also argues that the same evolution is taking place on the mainland. As long as the identity problem is not resolved, there is no certainty that free elections alone will help reduce polarization and lead to convergence among Taiwanese. Conversely, it can also be argued that the status quo is likely to prevail as most Taiwanese want neither independence nor reunification. But while nearly four out of five Taiwanese favour the status quo, support for reunification is declining steadily (Chu, 2001; Sheng, 2002).

From control to steering? Taiwanese society in the era of democratization

Issues of identity and political freedom were prominent throughout Taiwan's transition to democratic rule. At the same time, state–society relations evolved and affected both businesses and civil society organizations. Two main issues arise in this regard: is Taiwan pluralist or corporatist? Is Taiwanese society compliant or rebellious?

It has been argued that 'Corporatism's defining characteristics – state structuring, state subsidy, and state control – describe Taiwan's interest-group system well' (Rigger, 1996: 302). State structuring is defined here as 'a system of officially sanctioned, non-competitive, compulsory interest associations', while state control refers to 'state-imposed constraints on demand-making, leadership, and internal governance' (Rigger, 1996: 302). In contrast, in a pluralist system, 'groups of citizens organise themselves independently to pursue common interests; the state is merely a referee among these independent groups' (Rigger, 1996: 302).

In the early years of the KMT rule, Taiwanese society hardly enjoyed any autonomy. The state intervened strongly in the island's economy through state-owned enterprises, the import-substitution industrialization (ISI) model and a firm control of the labour movement. The party 'channelled emerging socio-economic interests into state-sponsored organisations' (Rigger, 1996: 302). In particular, 'some groups – including farmers, women, labour, and industrialists – even enjoyed reserved seats in legislative bodies. The regime made no secret of its intention to control these organisations' (Rigger, 1996: 302).

Leng (1996) argues that the dynamic changed after Chiang Ching-kuo decided to liberalize the regime. As a result,

> the democratisation process has acted as a catalyst for the split in the political elite and the convergence of technocrats and local interests, thus creating a dynamic civil society capable of resisting state intervention in both economic and political affairs.
>
> (Leng, 1996: 12)

While the gradual democratization that started in the 1950s and 1960s did not lead to any significant change in the corporatist structure set up by the KMT regime, the political liberalization of the late 1980s resulted in increased autonomy for both market and civil society organizations. This does not mean that the corporatist arrangements of the authoritarian era disappeared, but opportunities arose for non-state organizations to challenge government policies and/or establish a more favourable bargaining position. Examples include the increased autonomy of business associations (Leng, 1996) and the growing influence of social movements, in particular with regard to environment (Rigger, 1996).

Notwithstanding the leading role of the state in Taiwan's economic miracle, 'the most dynamic parts of the economy have generally been small and medium-sized enterprises (SMEs) which have few direct linkages with the state' (Lam and Clark, 1998: 120). Kuo (1995) emphasized that focusing on either the state or SMEs leads one to miss the key dimension of state–society interactions. 'The major reason for Taiwan's economic success in the past thirty years is the existence of strong cooperation between the state and business – not, as the statists have claimed, because of the existence of an autonomous state' (Kuo, 1995: 163).

As democracy matures and comes of age on the island, Taiwan's vibrant civil society increasingly reflects its political diversity. In particular, it was noted that

> One of the most significant transformations taking place in Taiwan since the 1980s has been the emergence of a demanding civil society. Being a demanding civil society, Taiwan has witnessed two distinguishable yet related social changes. One is the rise of a social movement sector within the non-governmental organizations, the other the self-transformation of many already well-established non-governmental organizations.
>
> (Hsiao, 1995: 239)

In an assessment of the strengths and weaknesses of Taiwanese civil society, though, it was recognized that 'the deepening of democracy in Taiwan has encouraged the growth of civil society and led to an explosion in the number of Taiwanese CSOs' (Lin, 2005: 92). But although civil society organizations evolve in an enabling environment and have a strong commitment to values, their structures remains weak (Lin, 2005). Taiwanese non-profit organizations can register either as foundations or as associations (Hsiao, undated) but the institutional framework in which civil society organizations operate still has a clear corporatist orientation. There is no unified regulatory framework for NPOs and the requirements depend on the field of activity. NPOs have to register with one of 13 government agencies, which retain a measure of discretion over the conditions attached (Hsiao, undated). In addition, as an association must have a minimum of 30 founding members,

> many chose to apply for establishing foundations simply because they wish to avoid losing control for having too many members. However, such alternative can be possible only if a required endowment is secured and available. Therefore, for those who lack the necessary funding to be required for setting up foundations are reluctantly to opt for the membership associations.
>
> (Hsiao, undated)

Requirements for registration are complex and sometimes confusing. In addition, it was found that 'in Taiwan, the formation of civil associations has often been encouraged by the government as a way of pursuing government objectives' (Feng, 1999: 326) and that 'the governing authority places more emphasis on the foundation's utility in helping the government with its duties than on the operational issues at the foundation, such as the integrity of board members' (Feng, 1999: 328–9). In spite of Taiwan's political liberalization and democratization, it is still too early to talk of the demise of corporatism and its replacement with open state–society relations in the pluralist sense.

How the state mobilizes non-state actors in external relations

Society was not allowed to participate in policy-making from the 1940s to the early 1980s. As the island's diplomatic isolation grew, the state started mobilizing non-state actors towards external policy goals.

Market organizations in Taiwan's external relations

Taiwanese companies were encouraged to contribute to the island's diplomatic efforts through investments in countries and regions which the government regarded as critically important, such as Southeast Asia and Central America. Taiwanese business tycoons, in particular in Southeast Asia, were found more effective than government envoys in reaching out to heads of states and decision-makers (Chen, 2002). However, the effectiveness of specific policies to enrol private companies in diplomatic efforts was not established.

For instance, the impact of the Go-South policy was limited. To boost Taiwanese investments in Southeast Asia, the government 'provided systematic financial, technical, organizational and informational assistance to entice more enterprises to invest in Southeast Asia, or help those which had already invested there' (Chen, 2002: 111). While the Taiwanese authorities tried to stem the flow of investment to the mainland, the policy was also viewed 'as a deliberate effort to strengthen Taiwan's economic diplomacy with Southeast Asian states' (Deng, 2000: 968). Taiwanese FDI to Southeast Asia kept rising until the 1997 financial crisis, but was found to be primarily motivated by comparative advantages and other business considerations. In particular,

> low-cost labor ranks at the top among the factors which motivate Taiwanese investment towards Southeast Asia. The market expansion motive is distant second, followed by the risk diversification concern, and the desire to obtain cheaper land in the host country.
>
> (Chen, 1998: 17)

Similarly, only one out of 59 small firms and three out of 51 large firms in a survey reported investing overseas at the urge of the Taiwanese government (Chen and Liu, 1998). In contrast, Taiwanese investments to the mainland kept soaring, although less than half of these investments were approved by the Taiwan government (Deng, 2000). Like Korean, Hong Kong or Singaporean companies, Taiwanese companies are attracted by the potential of the mainland market and low production costs, while China sees Taiwanese investments as a way to help promote reunification. In particular, official Taiwanese business associations enjoy a special status on the mainland (Ngo, 1995). Taiwanese entrepreneurs on the mainland have generally opposed policies that increased cross-strait tension.

Civil society organizations in Taiwan's external relations

Ahead of the 2000 presidential election, Chen Shui-bian announced that, if he was elected, a significant shift in Taiwan's foreign policy would occur. Declaring that the 'dollar diplomacy' of the past was bankrupt, he made the case for a diplomacy driven by human rights and unrestrained by Taiwan's status. In particular, he announced that NGOs would be encouraged to help expand Taiwan's diplomatic space. One of the reasons he mentioned is that 'NGOs advance international cooperation and peace' (*Taipei Times*, 18 August 2000).

Taiwanese NGOs were sometimes described as a bridge between the island and the mainland (Wang, 2000). But while some groups advocated closer ties with the PRC, others pushed for a more assertive stance. Taiwan's campaign to re-enter the United Nations is the result of civil society activism that developed after martial law was lifted in 1987. This civil society activism was naturally oppositional and helped shape the foreign policy agenda of the DPP (Näth, 1998).

Through the Foreign Affairs Institute, the Ministry of Foreign Affairs initially focused on 'training in topics such as cross-strait relations, international law and politics, negotiation, and the international role of non-governmental organisations' (Republic of China Yearbook Taiwan, 2002). The next step was the establishment of an NGO Affairs Committee to 'assist Taiwan's NGOs in their engagement of international NGO activities' (Republic of China Yearbook Taiwan, 2002). More specifically, the Committee advised and trained Taiwanese NGOs on ways and strategies to affiliate with UN-accredited INGOs. To this effect the MoFA approved numerous grants to Taiwan's NGOs to organize 'international events, meetings, and conferences in Taiwan or to travel to participate in such activities overseas' (Republic of China Yearbook Taiwan, 2002). In some cases the Ministry also 'facilitated visa processing for these activities' (Republic of China Yearbook Taiwan, 2002). As summarized by a legislator, 'NGOs have become Taiwan's "unofficial diplomats" in countries where we do not have ambassadors and representative offices' (*Taiwan News*, 11 June 2002).

NGO leaders in Taiwan, while welcoming the support pledged, nonetheless voiced their concerns. '"I hope the ministry can offer us substantial assistance by playing an assisting role rather than treating us with a sort of 'management mentality,'" said Shih Shin-min, a committee member and president of the Taiwan Environmental Protection Union' (*Taipei Times*, 3 October 2000). Similarly the chairwoman of the National Youth Commission, Lin Fang-mei, reportedly stated that 'Taiwan's NGOS should focus on their development as NGOs, not as instruments of the foreign ministry' (*Taipei Times*, 16 June 2001). Shifting the focus from material to physical instruments, another observer argued that

> If the ministry wants to assist the NGO community there is something very concrete it can do. It can ensure that visitors invited to Taiwan on NGO business are not delayed or denied entry due to any blacklist or being from 'an enemy state.' It is an interesting irony that the ministry harps on about 'what the foreign ministry can do to enhance Taiwan's international image' but in fact it does not do the few things within its power towards that end. One only needs to remember the denial of an entry visa to Nobel Peace Prize winner Jose Ramos Horta a couple of years ago to see that the ministry fails to do the things that it can to raise Taiwan's international image.
>
> (*Taipei Times*, 16 June 2001)

The internationalization of Taiwanese civil society organizations

One possible strategy is for Taiwanese NGOs to affiliate with international NGOs already in relations with the UN. Another strategy, mentioned by the NGO Committee, is to try and internationalize Taiwanese NGOs. As an example, the largest Taiwanese charity, the Buddhist Compassion Relief Tzu Chi Foundation, decided to

> unite its more than 100 branch offices around the world into a single organisation.... Once the new organisation is fully established, it plans to register with the United Nations as a non-governmental health organisation. Garnering the UN's official imprimatur would mean foreign nations are more likely to recognise and respect the group, and this in turn would facilitate the Tzu Chi Foundation's efforts to provide relief services around the world.
>
> (*Taiwan Headlines*, 22 November 1999)

As the number of possible candidates for such a strategy is very limited, the main thrust is to try and affiliate Taiwanese NGOs with international NGOs already accredited with the UN. How successful is Taiwan in its attempts to create the non-official diplomatic space it yearns for?

Taiwan was represented in 1,335 international organizations in 2006, against 1,752 for China and 1,327 for Hong Kong (Union of International Associations, 2007). Taiwan ranks fortieth for the number of international meetings it hosted in 2006. Taiwan hosted 21 NGO headquarters in 2006 and was ranked forty-fifth, just three places behind China. Taiwan, predictably, does not host the headquarters of a single intergovernmental organization, but neither do Hong Kong or China (Union of International Associations, 2007: 88). Taiwan's claims of isolation must therefore be put in perspective: although not part of the 200-member UN club, Taiwan consistently reaches the top 50 for key international socialization indicators.

In dynamic terms, Taiwan added 62 IO memberships from 2004 to 2006 and overtook Hong Kong, which added only 12 (Union of International Associations, 2007). Taiwan ranks forty-sixth globally, up from fiftieth two years ago. The number of principal secretariats of international organizations hosted by Taiwan was nearly unchanged in the 1990s – at around 30 – but rose to 55 in 2006. These are clearly important achievements, but the specific contribution of the government's NGO policy cannot be ascertained. Surveys ranking the motivations of NGOs would help clarify to what extent the MoFA influences NGOs' decisions on overseas networking and affiliations.

Overseas Taiwanese civil society organizations, such as the World Taiwanese Congress or the Formosan Association for Public Affairs (FAPA), are also of interest. The FAPA has become a 'world-wide, Washington headquartered, non-profit organization' and seeks to 'establish an independent and democratic country, and to join the international community' (Formosan Association for Public Affairs, undated). The association has endorsed Taiwan's UN bid, disseminates information regarding Taiwan's situation in the US and lobbies Congressmen. The FAPA stimulated the creation of a Congressional Taiwan Caucus (CTC), which had 150 members as of October 2005 (Formosan Association for Public Affairs, undated), up from 119 members as of 30 June 2003.

Concluding comments

This overview highlights that Taiwan's pariah status is the consequence of shifting alliances in the second part of the Cold War and Chiang Kai-shek's inflexibility. Taiwan appears to behave like a state, though one that sometimes portrays itself as an NGO or a functional entity for tactical purposes. Taiwanese non-state organizations were initially ignored by the state. As Taiwan's isolation grew while the island developed economically and matured politically, the state sought to involve non-state organizations in various ways to help expand Taiwan's diplomatic space. Taiwan's businesses often acted as informal ambassadors of the KMT regime. Later on, the DPP sought to enrol NGOs in diplomacy. Past corporatist arrangements, though still present, have given way to a more pluralist society.

This complex evolution is now studied in the cases of Taiwan's WHO campaign and Taiwan's medical and humanitarian aid programmes. The two case studies that follow highlight different aspects of Taiwan's position in global governance. Taiwan's WHO campaign is a prime example of how Taiwan uses the various components of governance to enhance its status globally. Taiwan seeks to expand and strengthen diplomatic ties through disaster relief and medical assistance, enrolling non-state agents in its efforts. Both case studies relate to state humanitarianism, i.e. the increasing use of humanitarian symbols and organizations by states as they seek to drive governance processes to their advantage in the global arena.

4 Taiwan's WHO campaign

Key governance elements

Introduction

Taiwan's bid to become an observer at the World Health Assembly was launched in 1997. The bid is analysed in line with the elements of governance (norms, actors, processes and outputs/outcomes) identified in Chapter 2. The elements are identified with regard to the WHO in general and in parallel to Taiwan's campaign to obtain observer status. As Taiwan is an irregular state, attention is paid in particular to the issues that make its bid problematic. The elements of governance systems identified in Chapter 2 provide a framework for such an analysis in this chapter. They are then brought together in Chapter 5 to provide a more comprehensive analysis of the campaign and Taiwan's dilemmas.

The World Health Organization was created in 1948 as the unitary arm of the United Nations in the field of health, in response to the shortcomings of previous attempts to tackle global health threats and concerns. Cooperation between nation-states on health issues was non-existent until the nineteenth century. As global trade and travel expanded, epidemic outbreaks of diseases endemic to tropical countries, primarily cholera, started spreading quickly to European countries, which had been spared so far. Both the speed of the steamship and the opening of the Suez Canal in 1869 drastically reduced the travel time between Asia and Europe (Siddiqi, 1995).

In response, European governments instituted quarantine measures in a rather anarchical way. The cholera pandemics that affected Europe in the 1830s and 1840s led to pressing calls for international cooperation, and the first International Sanitary Conference (ISC) was convened in Paris in 1851. The agenda of the conference was limited to cholera, plague and yellow fever.

The Paris Conference was followed by ten more conferences in the second half of the nineteenth century. As the cause of epidemic outbreaks had not yet been scientifically ascertained, diplomatic considerations prevailed over public health issues and physicians were sidelined. Echoing contemporary debates at the World Trade Organization, the major trading nations of the day, Britain and France, promoted the least trade-restrictive measures in order to protect their interests. Smaller European nations were not so enthusiastic. Persia and the Ottoman Empire resented being referred to as countries where epidemics originated. In short, state interests structured the field of international health cooperation, to the near exclusion of any other consideration.

As science progressed and the agents causing these epidemics were discovered in the last two decades of the nineteenth century, international health cooperation started developing on more scientific grounds. The decision to set up the first international health organization, the Office International d'Hygiène Publique (OIHP) [International Office of Public Hygiene], was taken at the eleventh conference in 1903.

The victors of the First World War decided that specialized international agencies should come under the firm control of the newly established League of Nations and that the OIHP should merge with the League Health Organization. Curiously, this never happened. Even though the OIHP had neither the necessary mandate nor the resources to tackle massive epidemics in the aftermath of the First World War, such as typhus and influenza, the organization successfully managed to fend off no less than four merger attempts. The OIHP even managed to outlive the League Health Organization, and eventually merged into the World Health Organization. Under the League system of governance, the decision-making processes of specialized agencies were closely associated with the League's core mission of peace-making activities. These agencies were affected by the League's growing irrelevance to international security in the 1930s (Siddiqi, 1995).

The founding members of the United Nations therefore decided to grant specialized agencies more institutional autonomy, but wanted the most prominent specialized agencies to agree to a framework of coordination under the Economic and Social Council (ECOSOC) to avoid overlapping mandates and duplication of efforts. WHO institutions were therefore designed to rectify earlier shortcomings in international health cooperation.

Governance norms: the WHO and Taiwan's bid for observer status

The norms adopted by the founding members of the WHO are reflected in its statutes. While the political dimension was present right from the beginning of international sanitary cooperation, the scientific dimension only emerged in the late nineteenth century. Founding members decided to give the WHO a wider mandate than the League Health Organization: a humanitarian dimension was added to political and scientific norms. The three main themes Taiwan harnesses in support of its observership bid reflect the three types of norms that structure the WHO's mandate: political, scientific/medical/technical and humanitarian.

Political norms and arguments

The founding members of the WHO defined health as 'a state of complete physical, mental and social well-being and not merely the absence of disease or infirmity' and stated that 'the health of all peoples is fundamental to the attainment of peace and security and is dependent upon the fullest co-operation of individuals and

States' (WHO, 2007: 1). Health thus defined has highly political ramifications. It is difficult to conceive of any field of human activity that would neither impact health nor be affected by health. The WHO's mandate lies at the intersection of three sets of norms: political, scientific/medical/technical, and humanitarian.

In addition to peace, security and cooperation, the WHO's constitution states that unequal development is a common danger, in particular because of communicable diseases. The WHO's constitution also emphasizes the need to 'establish and maintain effective collaboration with the United Nations, specialized agencies, governmental health administrations' and focus on 'the improvement of nutrition, housing, sanitation, recreation, economic or working conditions and other aspects of environmental hygiene' (WHO, 2007: 2).

One of Taiwan's main arguments is that the WHO should live up to its constitution as a universal body. How can the WHO be a universal organization if 23 million people in Taiwan are kept outside? The argument mirrors Taiwan's rationale to be readmitted to the United Nations. It is articulated around the points mentioned in Chapter 3, namely that Taiwan is a sovereign country with a significant population, territory and economic weight, which the PRC has never controlled. Taiwan denies that its participation would violate China's:

> First, in order to avoid the political issue of sovereignty, Taiwan is only seeking to become an *observer* in the WHA (rather than a full member) in its capacity as a 'health entity'. Second, there exist clear precedents for such observership both in the actual practice of the WHO and also based on the important world-wide trend towards inclusive participation in international fora.
>
> (Taiwan Ministry of Foreign Affairs, undated: 2)

Scientific/medical/technical norms and arguments

The WHO is mandated to facilitate and promote research, focus specifically on applied research and public health concerns, and establish international standards in various areas: teaching and training of health workers (Art. 2(o)), diagnostic procedures (Art. 2(t)), food, biological and pharmaceutical products (Art. 2(u)).

Taiwan argues that these issues lie at the core of the WHO's mission. Even where nations sit on opposite sides of a political dispute, Taiwan argues, they should cooperate to control and respond to epidemics, enhance research and medical progress, and disseminate techniques and treatments if they are to eradicate infectious diseases and achieve 'health for all'.

International health cooperation in the nineteenth century relied on quarantine, as the causes of infectious diseases were not ascertained. Quarantine gained prominence again as the SARS epidemic quickly spread across borders in 2003. China, Taiwan, Hong Kong, Singapore and Vietnam were most affected by the epidemic. Taiwan claimed that its exclusion from the WHO made the response to an unknown disease more difficult.

Taiwan argues that cooperation in medical research is needed for the general progress of mankind and that its exclusion from the WHO leads to a suboptimal outcome, as 'the PRC has never exercised any authority or jurisdiction over Taiwan's health care system, nor has the PRC contributed any part of its national budget to the health needs of Taiwan' (Taiwan Ministry of Foreign Affairs, undated: 8). In particular, Taiwan complained that it was not adequately informed about SARS diagnostic and treatment research. Taiwan also argues that its exclusion from the WHO hampers the dissemination of techniques and treatments and that other countries could benefit from its own experience if Taiwan was allowed to join the organization. Taiwan regularly emphasizes its own achievements including universal medical coverage, high life expectancy and low child mortality. Taiwan also insists that it was the first country to provide free and universal hepatitis B immunization for children. Taiwan also says it has been free of polio since 1985. Taiwan was not specifically declared polio-free by the WHO, as it is not a member state, but de facto recognized polio-free as part of China in 2000 (*Taipei Times*, 31 October 2000).

Referring to the lofty goal of 'health for all', Taiwan argues that its exclusion from the WHO is a denial of 'health for all Taiwanese'. Lastly, Taiwan claims that it was an active member of the organization from 1948 to 1972.

Humanitarian norms and arguments

The WHO's mandate specifies certain vulnerable groups in its constitution, including mothers and children, and the peoples of trust territories. In particular, the constitution's preamble insists that 'healthy development of the child is of basic importance'. The mandate is also defined with regard to specific circumstances, such as emergencies (Art. 2(d)). In such cases the WHO is mandated to bring appropriate aid and assistance 'upon the request of governments'.

Taiwan emphasizes the dual humanitarian dimension of its WHO bid. On the one hand, Taiwanese people suffer because they are excluded from the WHO. On the other hand, people in other countries suffer because Taiwan's exclusion makes it impossible to provide all the aid it could and would like to offer. As reported by a Taiwanese official in *The Lancet*,

> health officials and medical professionals in Taiwan have experienced great difficulties taking part in WHO and forums and workshops concerning the latest technologies in the diagnosis, monitoring and control of disease. … Because of this exclusion, Taiwan cannot develop adequate health-care policies and is in no position to learn the latest international advances in medical science. The ROC's health authorities have been denied the right to maintain normal contact with WHO, even in emergency cases involving contagious diseases. Nor can Taiwan take part in the work of such institutions as the FAO/WHO Codex Alimentarius Commission, a key organization whose mandate is to protect the health of consumers and promote the coordination of all food standards. Since Taiwan has been excluded from WHO, it is ineligible

> for assistance from WHO or its member states after an outbreak of disease, and Taiwanese officials are not allowed to visit pertinent countries to gain from their experience in disease control.
>
> (Tsai, 1999: 2157)

To illustrate the adverse impacts of exclusion, Taiwan focuses on three episodes: an epidemic of enterovirus 71 in 1998, the Chi-Chi earthquake in 1999 and SARS in 2003. To understand the structure of the argument, it is necessary to briefly describe these events.

Three illustrations of the fusion of norms

In 1998, Taiwan was struck by a large-scale outbreak of hand, foot and mouth disease. Most cases were children aged below six. Enterovirus 71 was identified as the agent. Since 1990, Taiwan operates a sentinel reporting system which includes sentinel physicians across the island, and teaching hospitals and regional hospitals for severe cases. In the 1998 enterovirus 71 outbreak, 818 sentinel physicians and 40 medical centres and regional hospitals reported 129,106 cases and 405 severe cases respectively (Ho *et al.*, 1999). The total number of cases in Taiwan was possibly ten times higher, as only one in ten physicians was included in the sentinel.

First recognized in 1969, enterovirus 71 has been identified in 12 outbreaks since. The very large number of cases in the 1998 outbreak in Taiwan puzzled epidemiologists, as enterovirus 71 had not been reported as affecting so many patients in previous outbreaks, such as in Bulgaria in 1975, Hungary in 1978 or Sarawak, Malaysia, in 1997. Of the 405 cases categorized as severe in the 1998 outbreak in Taiwan, 78 died, i.e. a fatality rate of 19.3 per cent. Enterovirus 71 returned in the following years following the same seasonal pattern: April–July, with a peak in June. In 1999, 35 severe cases were reported, nine of whom died. In 2000 and 2001 the fatality rate was 14.1 per cent, with 291 and 389 cases reported respectively.

Epidemics of hand, foot and mouth disease have been attributed to various viruses in the past, and in particular to enterovirus 71. But researchers writing on the 1997 Sarawak outbreak, which killed 29 children, noted that 'a large cluster of deaths resulting from a similar illness has been described in only one other instance, during an extensive outbreak of HFMD caused by EV71 in Taiwan in 1998' (Chan *et al.*, 2000: 681–2). This similarity, in the clinical presentation of fatal cases if not in the scale of the epidemic, was the basis for Taiwan's complaint.

> An example of the needless suffering this causes arose in 1998 when Malaysia experienced an outbreak of enterovirus. Taiwan was severely harmed because information about the epidemic was not made available to its officials in time for implementation of effective preventive measures.
>
> (Tsai, 1999: 2157)

Taiwan also complains that the WHO did not provide assistance when, on 21 September 1999, the island was struck by the most powerful earthquake in a century. More than 2,000 people died (*Reliefweb*, 29 November 1999). Although many countries immediately sent rescue teams or provided financial aid, Taiwan complained that its exclusion from the United Nations and specialized agencies led to delays. One specific complaint was that a Russian plane carrying relief goods, barred from flying over Chinese airspace, was delayed by ten hours (*Taipei Times*, 25 September 1999).

Other delays resulted from China's insistence that all international assistance, in particular a UNOCHA fact-finding and assessment mission, be cleared and specifically authorized by Beijing. Several countries, including Japan, reportedly waited for Beijing's approval. Taiwan scolded China for deliberately putting political considerations above the well-being of the Taiwanese people it claimed to represent. Taiwan also criticized the UN and the countries that felt obliged to ask for Beijing's permission.

In March 2003 the world was struck by a deadly form, hitherto unknown, of atypical pneumonia. Although SARS had probably been spreading for several months in South China, the world discovered the disease when the first case was identified in Hong Kong. China, Hong Kong, Taiwan and Singapore were the most affected countries and territories.

From 25 February to 16 June 2003, 3,032 cases of suspected or probable SARS were reported to the Centre for Disease Control of the Department of Health (Taiwan CDC). Among these cases, 664 were classified as probable SARS based on the WHO and CDC case definitions. Of those cases, 346 were confirmed as infected with the SARS coronavirus (Hsueh and Yang, 2003). During the first stage of the outbreak, the infection could be traced to travellers who had just returned from the mainland or Hong Kong, or had been in contact with index cases. During the second stage, from mid-April to mid-June, most of the cases 'occurred during a large nosocomial outbreak in a regional hospital in Taipei City and in subsequent inter-hospital spreads and intra-hospital transmission nationwide' (Hsueh and Yang, 2003: 829).

Of the 346 reported SARS patients, 73 died, i.e. a case fatality rate of 21.2 per cent. Of the deaths, 37 'were considered to have resulted directly from SARS' (Hsueh and Yang, 2003). As the epidemic swept through Asia, much attention was paid to developments in China, where information had been scarce. The Chinese authorities were criticized when it became clear that the real number of confirmed and suspected SARS cases in China was much higher than the number reported to the WHO.

While frontline medical workers everywhere struggled to contain the disease, which struck many of them, and researchers raced to identify its cause, much criticism was directed at health and hospital authorities across the region, in particular in Greater China. This was understandable as waves of nosocomial infections, in particular in Hong Kong, Taiwan and Singapore, hit doctors, nurses and patients alike. In Vietnam the course of the epidemic was atypical. After an initial outbreak in a hospital in Hanoi, where drastic isolation measures were immediately taken, no further infection was reported.

Taiwan argued that China's cover-up resulted in serious suffering on the island, which showed how little the Peoples' Republic cared for Taiwanese 'compatriots'. China was not just helpless, its actions were harmful. Taiwan's health authorities claimed that they did not have access to critical medical information that could have helped save lives in the acute phase of the epidemic. In particular, it was argued that because Taiwan

> was not able to get advice and practical support from the WHO in a timely manner – for example, on preventing hospital transmission and implementing in-hospital prevention measures – much energy has been misspent and the holes created by mistakes have yet to be plugged. Vietnam, in contrast, has far fewer resources of its own compared to Taiwan, but received a great deal of WHO help and was able to rapidly control the spread of the virus.
>
> (Lee, 2003)

Taiwan also blamed WHO headquarters in Geneva for failing to respond promptly to requests for help. While acknowledging that the WHO did send a team in May, authorities claimed that the WHO ignored previous requests for help from Taiwan's Department of Health in March (Taiwan Ministry of Foreign Affairs, undated). Taiwan also complained that the travel advisory issued against the island resulted in massive economic losses.

Immediate lessons from the analysis of norms

In all three episodes, Taiwan argued that China's actions and China's pressure on the UN and WHO made Taiwanese people's plight worse. Taiwan also uses the humanitarian argument in reverse mode when it argues that other countries are suffering as a result of Taiwan's exclusion from the WHO:

> The ROC has in recent years extended humanitarian and medical aid to various countries worldwide. Its government and its people have responded to appeals for emergency relief from countries that have been affected by natural disasters. Taiwan has demonstrated an excellent ability to conduct effective cooperation in aid and health operations overseas. Last year the ROC moved rapidly to provide support to the nations of Central America hit by hurricane Mitch; more recently it has offered substantial assistance to relieving the refugee crisis in Kosovo. Although Taiwan has shown that it is prepared to offer both technical and financial support to countries in need of improved health care, its exclusion from WHO hampers it in doing so. Nations that wish to collaborate with Taiwan and learn from its rapid improvements in health care over the past few decades are denied the correct channel through which to do it. Allowing Taiwan to participate in WHO would enable the country to contribute

> more easily to humanitarian health projects and in turn lessen suffering across the world.
>
> (Tsai, 1999: 2157)

It is difficult to link any particular WHO activity or programme to a single set of norms. All three aspects (political, scientific and humanitarian) are particularly enmeshed in the eradication paradigm. Eradication succeeded in the case of smallpox, and is arguably in sight for polio. But in the past two decades infectious diseases once thought to be good candidates for control if not eradication, such as tuberculosis and malaria, re-emerged and new ones such as AIDS emerged.

Eradication appears to have been the defining paradigm in an era when faith in scientific progress was yet to be shaken, the physical and budgetary requirements of public health were unquestioned, and the humanitarian concern for those most immediately at risk translated into unequivocal commitments of the international community. The culmination of the WHO's optimism was reflected in the 1978 Alma-Ata Declaration, which spelled out the objective of health for all by the year 2000. The purpose was to

> underline the fact that despite the ambitious proclamations enshrined in the WHO Constitution, large numbers of people and even whole countries, were not enjoying an acceptable standard of health. By the late 1970s nearly 1 billion people were living in poverty.
>
> (WHO, undated)

Over time, it became obvious that health for all would not be achieved by the year 2000. At the fifty-first World Health Assembly, members reframed the challenge as 'Health for all in the twenty-first century' and adopted the World Health Declaration:

> We recommit ourselves to strengthening, adapting and reforming, as appropriate, our health systems, including essential public health functions and services, in order to ensure universal access to health services that are based on scientific evidence, of good quality and within affordable limits, and that are sustainable for the future.
>
> (WHO, 1998a)

The norms and principles Taiwan invokes in support of its WHO bid derive from the same three streams: political, scientific/medical/technical and humanitarian. The main political norm Taiwan invokes is universality. With regard to scientific and technical norms, Taiwan emphasizes that the rationalization of public health efforts requires increased coordination between nations to help prevent, control and fight epidemics. From a humanitarian standpoint Taiwan argues that its exclusion from the WHO leads to increased suffering for both Taiwanese people and others.

The norms identified here are of course invoked by specific actors. The relevant actors are now introduced with regard to the WHO in general, before turning to those involved in Taiwan's campaign.

Governance actors: the WHO and Taiwan's bid for observer status

Status of participants in the WHO

Full membership of the World Health Organization is restricted to states, but 'shall be open to all states' (WHO, 2007: 3). States other than founding members 'may apply to become members and shall be admitted as members when their application has been approved by a simple majority vote of the Health Assembly' (WHO, 2007: 4). But participation is not restricted to states and the constitution stipulates that

> Territories or groups of territories which are not responsible for the conduct of their international relations may be admitted as Associate Members by the Health Assembly upon application made on behalf of such territory or group of territories by the Member or other authority having responsibility for their international relations.
>
> (WHO, 2007: 4)

Representatives of associate members, as in the case of full members, 'should be qualified by their technical competence in the field of health'. In addition, they 'should be chosen from the native population'. Territories currently enjoying associate member status include Puerto-Rico (since 1992), with the assent of the US, and Tokelau (since 1991), under the responsibility of New Zealand. Former associate members, including Southern Rhodesia, Papua New Guinea and Namibia, were admitted as full members after gaining independence. Besides members and associate members, the Constitution provides for the participation of other entities. In particular, the Health Assembly may invite

> any organization, international or national, governmental or non-governmental, which has responsibilities related to those of the Organization, to appoint representatives to participate, without right of vote, in its meetings or in those of the committees and conferences convened under its authority, on conditions prescribed by the Health Assembly; but in the case of national organizations invitations shall be issued only with the consent of the Government concerned.
>
> (WHO, 2007: 6).

In addition, specific provisions apply at the regional level:

> Territories or groups of territories within the region, which are not responsible for the conduct of their international relations and which are not associate

> members, shall have the right to be represented and to participate in regional committees. The nature and extent of the rights and obligations of these territories or groups of territories in regional committees shall be determined by the Health Assembly in consultation with the member or authority having responsibility for the international relations of these territories and with the member states in the region.
>
> (WHO, 2007: 12)

The rights and obligations of associate members and other territories were primarily defined by the first and second Health Assemblies in resolutions WHA1.80 and WHA2.103. Associate members have the right to participate,

> without vote in the deliberations of the Health Assembly and its main committees [and] with vote and to hold office in other committees or sub-committees of the Assembly, except the General Committee, the Committee on Credentials and the Nominations Committee.
>
> (WHO, 2007: 19)

They also have the right to 'propose items for inclusion in the provisional agenda of the Assembly [and] submit proposals to the Executive Board [but] shall not be eligible for membership on the Board' (WHO, 2007: 19–20).

The rights and obligations of associate members and other territories in regional organizations were defined by the Second Health Assembly in 1949 and the participants resolved that 'associate members shall have all rights and obligations in the regional organizations, with the exception that they will have no vote in plenary meetings of the regional committee, nor in subdivisions dealing with finance or constitutional matters' (WHO, 2007: 21).

In addition, it was resolved that the same rights shall apply in the case of territories not responsible for the conduct of their international relations and not associate members 'subject to consultation between the states members in a region and the members or other authority having responsibility for the international relations of these territories' (WHO, 2007: 21). Thus the Constitution of the World Health Organization and resolutions made by the first two Health Assemblies clearly defined three categories of participants at the regional level: members, associate members, and other territories not responsible for the conduct of their international relations.

In contrast, observer status is mentioned neither in the Constitution nor in resolutions of the Health Assembly. It only appears in the rules of procedure of the World Health Assembly. Rule 3 stipulates that

> the Director-General may invite States having made application for membership, territories on whose behalf application for associate membership has been made, and States which have signed but not accepted the Constitution to send observers to sessions of the Health Assembly.
>
> (WHO, 2007: 123)

Rule 47 stipulates that

> observers of invited non-Member States and territories on whose behalf application for associate membership has been made may attend any open meetings of the Health Assembly or any of its main committees. They may, upon the invitation of the President, and with the consent of the Health Assembly or committee, make a statement on the subject under discussion. Such observers shall have access to non-confidential documents and to such other documents as the Director-General may see fit to make available. They may submit memoranda to the Director-General, who shall determine the nature and scope of their circulation.
>
> (WHO, 2007: 133)

These rules of procedure focus on the case of territorial authorities, which are in the process of applying for either membership as a state, or associate membership with the agreement of the member state responsible for the international relations of the candidate. But they do not spell out the rules applicable to other organizations, 'international or national, governmental or non-governmental', referred to in Art. 18(h) of the Constitution.

In practice, observer status was granted over time to various entities, which do not necessarily conform to the regulatory stipulations mentioned above. Currently Palestine, the Holy See, the Sovereign Order of Malta, the International Committee of the Red Cross (ICRC) and the International Federation of Red Cross and Red Crescent Societies (IFRC) are invited as de facto permanent observers. There is no clear legal basis for the last three, but the Director-General in practice considers that it is his prerogative to invite such organizations to send observers and decide on the conditions attached without consulting the Health Assembly (Burci and Vignes, 2004). In addition,

> It is extremely significant that the Director-General, when issuing invitations, has deliberately avoided making any reference to 'observers status'. These observers are invited on a regular basis, but *de jure* the status of permanent observer has never existed in the WHO, this status existing only de facto.
>
> (Burci and Vignes, 2004: 38)

Observers can broadly be divided in two categories: 'territorial' and 'universal'. Palestine primarily defends the interests of Palestinian people even in the absence of clear statehood. In contrast, the Vatican, the Sovereign Order of Malta and the Red Cross do not defend the rights of people from a particular territory.

In addition to members, associate members and observers, the WHO encourages the participation of non-state actors to promote public health (WHO, 2002a). In 2001 the WHO launched the Civil Society Initiative (CSI) to 'identify and develop propositions for more effective and useful interfaces and relationships between civil society and the WHO' (Brundtland, 2001).

Grappling with a complex issue, the WHO/CSI recognized that there were many types of civil society organizations, that NGOs were just one kind of CSOs and that the boundaries between state, market and civil society were unclear. The WHO/CSI nonetheless emphasized 'the importance of differentiating between non-state actors with commercial or market interests and those without such interests' and recommended 'that market links or interests be transparent to WHO, particularly in the organization's normative and policy role' (WHO, 2002b: 5).

Acknowledging divisions and conflicting views within civil society, the discussion paper suggested that the WHO sort through CSOs according to the scope of potential collaboration: global, technical or institutional. The next step was a review of the existing policy. Civil society organizations were defined as non-state, non-profit, voluntary organizations. Distinguishing state from non-state organizations is sometimes problematic, as states may set up and fund NGOs/CSOs. Delineating market and non-market entities is also difficult, as firms can set up and fund non-profit organizations to represent their interests.

The organs and structure of the WHO

The WHO's main organs are the Assembly, the Executive Board and the Secretariat. The World Health Assembly is the supreme decision-making body of the organization. It determines its policies, appoints the Director-General, supervises the financial policies of the organization, reviews and approves the proposed programme budget and the reports and activities of both the Executive Board and the Director-General. The Assembly has the power to

> promote and conduct research in the field of health by the personnel of the Organization, by the establishment of its own institutions or by co-operation with official or non-official institutions of any Member with the consent of its Government ... establish such other institutions as it may consider desirable [and] take any other appropriate action to further the objective of the Organization.
>
> (WHO, 2007: 6)

The Executive Board 'shall exercise on behalf of the whole Health Assembly the powers delegated to it by that body' (WHO, 2007: 9). The Board is composed of 32 members elected for three-year terms. To ensure an equitable geographical distribution, 'no less than three [members] shall be elected from each of the regional organizations established' (WHO, 2007: 8). The main Board Meeting, held in January, adopts the agenda for the forthcoming Health Assembly. The Executive Board holds another meeting immediately after the Health Assembly. The Board gives effect to the decisions and policies of the Health Assembly and generally facilitates its work. In particular, the Board can

> authorize the Director-General to take the necessary steps to combat epidemics, to participate in the organization of health relief to victims of a

> calamity and to undertake studies and research the urgency of which has been drawn to the attention of the Board by any Member or by the Director-General.
>
> (WHO, 2007: 9)

The Secretariat employs around 8,000 experts and support staff at headquarters, in the six regional offices and in member countries. The Director-General is appointed by the Health Assembly on the nomination of the Executive Board. The Director-General 'shall be *ex-officio* Secretary of the Health Assembly, of the Board, of all commissions and committees of the Organisation and of conferences convened by it. He may delegate these functions' (WHO, 2007: 9). Art. 35 and Art. 37 respectively emphasize the 'internationally representative character of the Secretariat' and the 'international character of the Director-General and the staff' (WHO, 2007: 10).

Notwithstanding the emphasis on its international character, the organization has been decentralized since its creation. One reason is that the pre-existing regional Pan-American Health Organization was reluctant to a full merger. There are currently six regional offices: Europe, Africa, the Americas, Southeast Asia, Middle East and Western Pacific. Each regional organization 'shall be an integral part of the Organization in accordance with this Constitution [but also] consist of a regional committee and a regional office' (WHO, 2007: 12) and 'the head of the regional office shall be the Regional Director appointed by the Board in agreement with the regional committee' (WHO, 2007: 13). In practice, this means that regional directors are elected by the region's member states.

In addition to statutory organs, two mechanisms represent an important part of the WHO's operational capacity: WHO collaborating centres, and the Global Outbreak Alert and Response Network. WHO collaborating centres are national institutions selected by the Director-General to help implement WHO programmes and strengthen institutional capacity. The Global Outbreak Alert and Response Network, launched in 1997 and formally set up in 2000, pools technical and operational resources to respond to epidemic outbreaks. It includes

> scientific institutions in Member States, medical and surveillance initiatives, regional technical networks, networks of laboratories, United Nations organizations (e.g. UNICEF, UNHCR), the Red Cross (International Committee of the Red Cross, International Federation of Red Cross and Red Crescent Societies and national societies) and international humanitarian non-governmental organizations (e.g. Médecins sans Frontières, International Rescue Committee, Merlin and Epicentre). Participation is open to technical institutions, networks and organizations that have the capacity to contribute to international outbreak alert and response.
>
> (WHO, 2006a)

States in Taiwan's WHO bid

The actors and organizations involved in Taiwan's campaign mirror the categories described in the theoretical framework and referred to by the World Health

Organization: states, markets and civil society. The Taiwanese government leads Taiwan's efforts to join the WHO. The campaign involves the Ministry of Foreign Affairs and, to a lesser extent, the Department of Health. While decisions are made in Taipei, implementation relies primarily on Taiwan's diplomatic missions. Taiwan has two diplomatic missions in Geneva. The diplomatic mission involved in the WHO campaign is the Taipei Cultural and Economic Delegation. In 2002, an advisor to the Ministry of Health was posted in Geneva to coordinate the campaign. Taiwan's diplomatic missions elsewhere, in particular in the US, also play an important role.

Taiwan's official diplomatic allies have been involved in one or more of the following ways:

- Written to the Director-General of the World Health Organization to request that Taiwan's application for observer status be included in the agenda of the World Health Assembly.
- Spoken up in favour of Taiwan at a General Committee meeting of the World Health Assembly, during a plenary session of the Assembly or at an Executive Board meeting.
- Voted in favour of including Taiwan's application for observer status in the agenda of the fiftieth World Health Assembly and/or of the fifty-seventh World Health Assembly.

Supporters of Taiwan's WHO bid generally endorse Taiwan's UN bid too. Interestingly, not all of Taiwan's diplomatic allies have supported the WHO bid. Conversely, support has also come from countries with unofficial ties to Taiwan, including the US, Japan and EU member countries. The US Congress and the European Parliament have clearly endorsed Taiwan's bid, while Western governments were long reluctant to officially endorse Taiwan's bid. In 2004, though, during the first meeting of the General Committee of the Health Assembly, the US delegate noted that

> The advancement of global public health required Taiwan to have appropriate access to, participation in, and interaction with WHO, including in the Health Assembly. Taiwan had much experience to offer, but would also benefit through observer status, so improving the effectiveness of international public health measures. Taiwan did not qualify to be a Member of WHO, but the Health Assembly should distinguish between full membership and observership, and not hinder legitimate interaction with WHO.
>
> (WHO, 2004a: 6)

Conversely, most states oppose Taiwan's bid and support China's position. As Taiwan's attempts to break isolation in the global arena and its apparent or suspected moves towards independence are among Beijing's top concerns, it would be difficult to list all of China's state organizations involved in the campaign or to find any that never said anything on the issue. Close allies, including Pakistan and

Cuba, have consistently been at the forefront of the defence of China's position in the World Health Assembly.

Non-state actors in Taiwan's campaign

Taiwanese companies contributed to the island's diplomatic efforts in the 1990s, as highlighted in Chapter 3. The government encouraged Taiwanese businesses to invest in certain countries and regions, generating both goodwill and informal contacts. While such investments may indirectly boost Taiwan's WHO bid by bolstering diplomatic alliances, some companies have taken a more direct approach. Infinity Air, a little-known aviation company based in California and run by Taiwanese-Americans, approached the WHO with an offer to contribute US$1 million to a SARS research project. Initially, no political conditions were spelled out, but it turned out eventually that Infinity Air wanted the WHO to organize face-to-face meetings between Taiwanese and mainland officials (personal communication from a WHO officer, 17 June 2003).

While advancing their interests through NGOs, some business groups may also help support Taiwan's WHO bid. One example is the Foundation of Medical Professionals Alliance in Taiwan (FMPAT), a Taiwanese umbrella organization which actively supports Taiwan's WHO bid. The FMPAT, 'believing that the level of Taiwan's clinical-trial technology must be raised to prepare for a global boom in biotechnology … initiated a series of clinical-research seminars' (*Free China Journal*, 21 March 2003). The FMPAT also 'took part in the International Conference on Harmonization of Technical Requirements for Registration of Pharmaceuticals for Human Use', with a view to 'tout Taiwan's development as a pharmaceutical centre in the Asia-Pacific region' (*Free China Journal*, 21 March 2003). But the FMPAT focuses primarily on the WHO campaign, lobbies NGOs, governments and businesses and sponsors training sessions on international health and diplomacy. According to Lin Shih-chia, its executive director, 'ultimately, most of our efforts fall on helping Taiwan join the WHO' (*Free China Journal*, 21 March 2003).

The influence of Taiwanese businesses may not be limited to the island's political arena. In a House of Commons debate, the hon. Tom Cox, co-chairman of the all-party British-Taiwanese group, sought 'the views of the British government and their attitude to Taiwan's request for observer status within WHO', noting that 'Taiwan has been and is a major investor in this country' (United Kingdom Parliament, 2000). In his response, the Minister of State, Foreign and Commonwealth Office, John Battle, acknowledged that 'we have attracted almost 85 per cent of Taiwan's total investment in the European Union' (United Kingdom Parliament, 2000).

Various categories of NGOs have been involved to some degree in Taiwan's campaign. A core group of international medical associations publicly supports Taiwan's WHO bid, including the World Medical Association (WMA), the International Pharmaceutical Federation (IPF), the International Council of Nursing (ICN) and the International Paediatrics Association (IPA), (*Taipei Times*, 19 May

2003a). Taiwan is a long-standing member of the WMA, which represents more than eight million physicians worldwide. WMA members had reservations about China's application because of medical ethics concerns, in particular with regard to organ transplants. The Chinese Medical Association was admitted in 1989, but their membership lapsed two years later because they failed to pay membership fees. The Chinese Medical Association was readmitted in 1997 (World Medical Association, 1997). Board members of the World Medical Association and the World Surgeons' Association have included Taiwanese doctors and surgeons.

Taiwanese medical NGOs strongly support the WHO bid. In particular, the Taiwan International Medical Alliance (TIMA), founded in January 2001, seeks to 'promote Taiwan's participation in the World Health Organisation' (Taiwan International Medical Alliance, 2003) and unite Taiwan's medical organizations. Overseas Taiwanese NGOs, in particular the FAPA (see Chapter 3) also play a role. The FAPA closely monitors the State Department's actions in support of Taiwan's WHO bid and repeatedly pressed for more stringent legislation with regard to the reporting obligations of the State Department to Congress on the issue.

Driven by various norms and interests, the actors involved in Taiwan's observership bid are as diverse as those involved with the WHO. How do these actors interact in terms of global health governance, and in particular in the case of Taiwan's campaign?

Governance processes: the WHO and Taiwan's bid for observer status

Governance processes as defined in Chapter 2 in terms of linking arrangements and policy instruments are addressed here. State-to-state interactions are discussed first before turning to state–civil society interactions.

State-to-state interactions

State-to-state interactions within WHO are defined statutorily and carried out through the World Health Assembly, the Executive Board and the Secretariat. This framework constrains Taiwan's efforts to be admitted as an observer. As Taiwan cannot officially participate in the Health Assembly, Taiwan relies on others to speak on its behalf. Taiwan's diplomatic allies sitting on the WHO's board can raise the issue in January, as board members 'prepare the provisional agenda of each regular session of the Assembly after consideration of proposals submitted by the Director-General' (WHO, 2007: 123).

Any proposal by a Member State or Associate Member for the inclusion of an agenda item 'shall reach the Director-General not later than 10 weeks before the commencement of the session' (WHO, 2007: 155). The Director-General has the right to 'recommend the deferral or exclusion' of such proposals, on condition that 'the provisional agenda shall contain an explanation for such recommendation' (WHO, 2007: 155). This is a hurdle for Taiwan's allies, as the Director-General enjoys some measure of discretionary power. A second hurdle is that 'in adopting its agenda, the Board may decide to add to, delete from, or amend, the provisional agenda and any supplement thereto' (WHO, 2007: 156). In practice, the proposal to invite Taiwan as an observer never made it to the agenda of the Executive Board.

Next, the Board must 'include in the provisional agenda of each regular session of the Health Assembly *inter alia* any item proposed by a Member or by an Associate Member' (WHO, 2007: 123). However, the proposal to invite Taiwan as an observer was first introduced as a supplementary item. A supplementary item

> may be added to the agenda during any session, if upon the report of the General Committee the Health Assembly so decides, provided that the request for the inclusion of the supplementary item reaches the Organization within six days from the day of the opening of a regular session.
>
> (WHO, 2007: 125)

At the fiftieth World Health Assembly the proposal was made to include a supplementary agenda item to invite the Republic of China (Taiwan) to participate as an observer in the World Health Assembly (WHO, 1997). Although the General Committee of the Assembly recommended not to include this item in the agenda, the President asked for comments from members.

In a lengthy debate, the proposal was supported by Nicaragua, Dominica, Senegal, Gambia, the Solomon Islands, Swaziland, Grenada, République Centrafricaine, El Salvador, Saint Vincent and the Grenadines and the Dominican Republic, all Taiwan's diplomatic allies. In contrast, the delegates from Pakistan, Côte d'Ivoire, Guinée, Argentina, Cuba, Nepal, Myanmar, Kiribati, Egypt and Papua New Guinea spoke against the proposal (WHO, 1997).

Sovereignty was the only argument invoked by China's allies. The question of China's representation in the UN system had been settled long ago, they said. So there was no point wasting time, as mentioned by the delegate of Pakistan. The matter was an internal affair to be handled by the PRC, as noted by the delegate of Cuba (WHO, 1997).

The arguments put forward by Taiwan's supporters were more diverse. Of the 11 delegates who spoke in favour of Taiwan, seven mentioned that health is an inalienable right (Gambia, Solomon Islands, Swaziland, Grenada, République Centrafricaine, El Salvador and the Dominican Republic). As health for all is an intrinsic right and a goal stated by the WHO, the delegates of these countries said, the Republic of China cannot be excluded (WHO, 1997).

Six delegates specifically mentioned Taiwan's medical aid to developing countries (Nicaragua, Gambia, the Solomon Islands, Grenada, République Centrafricaine, Saint Vincent and the Grenadines). Noting that the Republic of China helped countries less fortunate than themselves, the delegate of Grenada stressed the need to maximize available resources. The delegate of Nicaragua emphasized that Taiwan not only promised but delivered aid (WHO, 1997).

Finally, four countries (Dominica, Senegal, the Solomon Islands and Swaziland) stated in nearly identical terms that contagious diseases know no boundaries.

Fighting them required the cooperation of all countries. The delegate of Dominica pointed out that outbreaks of disease originating from Taiwan could affect many countries around the world (WHO, 1997).

On each side, some delegates accused the other side of unnecessarily politicizing what they said should remain a purely medical or humanitarian issue. Also on each side, there were delegates who cast the issue as primarily political. In the end, the President ruled that a roll call vote would take place, as per WHO statutes. 128 members voted for the General Committee's recommendation not to include in the Assembly's agenda the proposal in favour of granting the Republic of China (Taiwan) observer status, whereas 19 voted against, and five abstained. Though not discussed as an agenda item, the proposal nonetheless kept the Assembly busy for several hours.

Interestingly, three of Taiwan's official diplomatic allies abstained (Costa Rica, the Bahamas and Panama) and four were absent (Saint-Kitts-and-Nevis, Saint Lucia, the Marshall Islands and Nauru). South Africa, still officially an ally at the time, and Belize, which later established official diplomatic links with Taiwan, voted against the proposal.

In subsequent years, an arrangement was found to avoid similarly lengthy debates and roll call votes: two countries would be invited to speak in the plenary in support of Taiwan's application, whereas China and one of its allies would speak against the proposal. The matter would then be closed. This scenario was repeated every year from 1998 to 2003.

In 2004, though, the Chinese representative could not prevent a debate, as Taiwan's allies demanded a vote. The debate and the vote lasted until the evening and the session of the first day was closed before the Director-General could deliver his annual address. Taiwanese officials were upbeat. Though the proposal was defeated by 133 votes to 25, the voting record was more favourable to Taiwan than the 128–19 tally in 1997. In addition, Taiwan's Deputy Foreign Minister Michael Kau noted that 'the number of WHA committee members who spoke out for Taiwan increased from seven last year to 16 this year' (*Free China Journal*, 28 May 2004), although he conceded that the number of delegates who spoke against Taiwan also rose, from 27 to 31. More importantly, for the first time the United States and Japan voted in favour of Taiwan's application.

The US Congress has passed bills supporting Taiwan's bid since 1999 (*Taipei Times*, 17 May 2004a). As the State Department showed little enthusiasm and support for Taiwan's WHO bid, the Congress passed increasingly binding resolutions. In 2002 and 2003, legislation was unanimously passed by both houses of Congress and signed by President George W. Bush. Finally, on 21 April 2004, the US House of Representatives resolved by a 416–0 vote to 'introduce a resolution on the floor of the World Health Assembly … in support of Taiwan's participation in the World Health Organisation with observer status' (Tkacik, 2004).

> In a statement on the signing of the bill into law, Bush said that the US fully supports the participation of Taiwan in the work of the WHO, including

> observer status. 'The United States has expressed publicly its firm support for Taiwan's observer status and will continue to do so,' Bush said.
>
> (*Taipei Times*, 16 June 2004)

The bill directs the Secretary of State to submit a yearly, non-confidential report to Congress detailing the measures taken to help Taipei gain observer status (*Taipei Times*, 16 June 2004). Reinforcing the legislative process, then US Secretary of Health and Human Services Tommy Thompson spoke publicly, and every year more forcefully, in favour of Taiwan. In 2002, Thompson spoke in favour of Taiwan during the annual conference of the World Medical Association and in 2003 at the World Health Assembly. As SARS was on everyone's mind, he insisted that global health cooperation was essential to fight epidemics. Ahead of the Assembly, the US urged the WHO to 'accommodate Taiwan in its health network', though this 'did not mean it supported the inclusion of Taiwan's observer status bid in the assembly agenda' (*Taipei Times*, 20 May 2003).

This led the Taiwanese Ministry of Foreign Affairs to hope that in 2004 Thompson would speak three times: at the General Committee, at the plenary of the Health Assembly, and 'after the Health Assembly when the EU is slated to explain why it had collectively voted in opposition to Taiwan's application' (*Taipei Times*, 17 May 2004b). During the Assembly Thompson stated that 'the United States of America fully supports the participation of Taiwan in the work of WHO, including observer status for Taiwan at the Health Assembly' (WHO, 2004c: 32) but cautioned that

> we do not support membership because Taiwan does not qualify to be a member of WHO. The people of Taiwan deserve to have an opportunity to observe. The Health Assembly makes a distinction between membership and observership and should not deny Taiwan's legitimate interaction with WHO.
>
> (WHO, 2004c: 33)

The intensity of Thompson's support for Taiwan's cause may have been related in part to his long-lasting friendship with Lee Ming-liang, a former director-general of Taiwan's Department of Health (interview with Peter Chang, 9 June 2004). When Lee paid his counterpart a visit in 2002, this was 'hailed as the first instance of a Taiwanese government official being welcomed into the office of an official of the US executive branch in 30 years' (*Taipei Times*, 17 May 2004a).

Taiwanese observers hoped that the gradual shift in the US position would have a positive impact on the position of its allies including Canada, Japan and European countries. The European Parliament expressed support for Taiwan and MPs formed Taiwan caucuses or friendship groups in the parliaments of several European countries but European governments do not support Taiwan's bid.

State–civil society interactions at the WHO

The issue of WHO–NGO relations was first broached in 1948 during the first World Health Assembly. The principles governing these relations were subsequently amended, and eventually codified in 1987 (WHO, 2001a). Separately, the WHO worked on a set of guidelines for interaction with commercial enterprises to achieve health outcomes, in order to prevent potential conflicts of interest. This document stated that such guidelines 'can also apply to a variety of other institutions including state-run enterprises, associations representing commercial enterprises, foundations not at arms length from their sponsors, and other non-profit organisations' (WHO, 2001b: 2).

The 1987 Principles address both formal and informal interactions between the WHO and NGOs/CSOs. The WHO's official relations are restricted to INGOs (International Non-Governmental Organizations). As of July 2002, 189 organizations were in official relations with the WHO. The drawn-out and highly bureaucratic process includes the drafting of a joint programme and a three-year plan. It must then be endorsed by the Executive Board. While most of these organizations specifically focus on medical and public health issues, the WHO is also in official relations with INGOs with a broader mandate, provided they focus primarily on health issues.

Other interactions were deemed informal. The review process established that at headquarter level 45 per cent of WHO relations with NGOs were official, and 55 per cent informal. The main difference is that NGOs in official relations can participate in the World Health Assembly or Executive Board meetings.

In its assessment, the WHO acknowledged that NGOs/CSOs contributed to policy definition and implementation and 'addressed sensitive issues that the WHO, as an intergovernmental organisation, may not be in a position to address for political reasons' (WHO, 2002c: 13). NGOs/CSOs were also viewed as better equipped to reach out to local communities. The WHO recognized that cooperating with NGOs/CSOs makes its work 'more visible and transparent and contributes towards actively building public accountability within the context of the widening UN framework for governance in global policy' (WHO, 2002c: 13).

CSOs criticized the WHO for its lack of transparency, noting information and communication gaps. The WHO acknowledged that it was ill-equipped to distinguish between organizations primarily guided by public interest and those promoting commercial interests. Conflicts of interest were not clearly defined. Lastly, the WHO acknowledged that its own accreditation procedures were lengthy, onerous and rigid, and did not provide the organization with updated information on the governance and funding of accredited CSOs/NGOs. In conclusion of the review process, the WHO/CSI recommended to:

1 Stick to the established definition of NGOs as non-state, non-profit, voluntary organizations.
2 Establish an accreditation policy for NGO participation in WHO governing bodies based on the following criteria: competence in a field of activity

relevant to the WHO's work, established structure, international scope and transparency.

3 Define a collaboration policy between the WHO Secretariat and NGOs to energize collaborations on the basis of reciprocity and transparency, and clarify how the WHO could support member states in their work with civil society.
4 Request NGOs seeking accreditation and/or collaboration to agree with the WHO's constitution and disclose their interests.

Discussing the proposals at their January 2003 meeting, WHO board members disagreed on three points. First, the issue of member states' control over the accreditation process was raised by the representative of China. He noted the lack of objective criteria to assess the competence of an NGO beyond the information provided by the applicant. He asked how the suitability of such collaboration would be assessed, and whether the final decision would be taken by the World Health Assembly or the Executive Board. The proposal submitted to the fifty-sixth World Health Assembly included these points and mentioned the requirement of demonstrated competence in a field of activity related to the work of the WHO.

Second, the representation of national NGOs. Several board members, led by Brazil, criticized the proposal that only INGOs be accredited with the WHO at headquarter level. Community-based NGOs in developing countries could contribute significantly to WHO policy-making and were closer to the needs of the people than those in the North, yet had fewer resources at their disposal, Brazil said. National NGOs should not be excluded from accreditation. The US delegate emphasized that national NGOs could join international federations to gain accreditation, and that care should be taken to ensure that the WHO's administrative burden at HQ level be minimized. The proposal submitted to the fifty-sixth Health Assembly stated that the membership and/or activities of NGOs applying for accreditation must be international in scope (WHO, 2003a).

Third, the distinction between for-profit and non-profit organizations, linked to the issue of conflicts of interests, was hotly debated. Several members mentioned that WHO interactions with the for-profit sector were legitimate but should be transparent. In particular, business interests should not disguise as NGOs. In response, the US delegate stated that conflicts of interest affected nearly everyone, including WHO member states, most EB members, NGO board members and non-profit organizations that did not report funding from private businesses in a transparent way. In defence of the for-profit sector, the US delegate stated that 'there were many non-profit organisations that did not always have the best interests of public health at heart, governments included' (WHO, 2003b). On this point the proposal submitted to the fifty-sixth World Health Assembly remained somewhat evasive and simply stated that an NGO seeking accreditation must 'be non-profit in nature' and 'disclose information on its objectives, structure, membership of executive body, field of activity and source of financing' (WHO, 2003a). The draft mentioned that collaboration with

NGOs 'shall be designed to avoid any conflicts of interests', but fell short of defining specifically what constitutes a conflict of interest.

Having worked hard on this compromise, WHO members were taken by surprise when China came up with its own draft during the Health Assembly, introducing substantive changes. First, China argued that the policy should only apply to international NGOs, defined by the international scope of their structure, in addition to membership and/or activities. Second, the WHO needed to follow its own rules and seek the consent of the government concerned before interacting with a national NGO. Finally, China insisted that INGOs could only participate in regional meetings at the invitation of the Regional Director.

These amendments were obviously intended to restrict, control and closely monitor working relations between the WHO and NGOs and represented a setback for those eager to see the WHO move towards less bureaucratic and more substantive relations with NGOs. An emergency meeting was convened to try and paper over these differences. Most participants, while regretting the abrupt change in China's position, were reluctant to hastily draft a compromise, given the importance and long-term implications of the policy, in spite of China's attempts to rush this through (personal communication of a WHO officer, Geneva, 18 June 2003). To the dismay of many, the NGO policy was withdrawn from the Assembly's agenda. Five years on, the official WHO policy vis-à-vis non-state actors, whether non-profit or for-profit, remains unchanged.

State–civil society interactions in Taiwan's WHO bid

Many civil society organizations are involved in Taiwan's WHO campaign. In growing numbers, Taiwanese supporters fly to Geneva every year to support Taiwan's bid. As reported by the *Taipei Times*,

> hundreds of Taiwanese from medical associations in Taiwan, Japan, North America, Europe and members of the Federation of Taiwanese Associations in Europe, as well as of the World Taiwanese Chambers of Commerce, have descended on Geneva for the week-long World Health Assembly meeting.
>
> (*Taipei Times*, 13 May 2002)

The President of the Taiwan Medical Association, Wu Yung-tung, reported that the number of members of his association who came to show support 'increased six-fold this year' (*Taipei Times*, 13 May 2002). The executive director of the Foundation of the Medical Professionals Alliance (FMPAT) said he was 'very thrilled to see that we no longer have only one group supporting the move' (*Taipei Times*, 13 May 2002). Standard events during the week of the Health Assembly include the unfurling of 'Taiwan for WHO' banners by Taiwanese activists at Place des Nations in the heart of Geneva's international enclave.

The enthusiasm of medical professionals for the campaign is understandable, as they started it. The Foundation of the Medical Professionals Alliance was one of the many civil society organizations created after the martial law was lifted. The foundation's main objective is Taiwan's participation in WHO (*Free China Journal*, 21 March 2003). The foundation forced the government to launch Taiwan's WHO bid, even though the Ministry of Foreign Affairs, which launched its own bid for UN membership in 1993, was initially reluctant (interview with Peter Chang, 9 June 2004). According to Wu Shuh-min, executive director of the Foundation of the Medical Professionals Alliance, 'while foreign ministry officials were rather cool to us when we were here for the first time in 1997 … we are now enjoying an increasingly closer relationship with the foreign ministry' (*Taipei Times*, 13 May 2002).

In contrast, not all Taiwanese humanitarian organizations show similar enthusiasm but Taiwanese diplomats routinely encourage them to help friendly countries respond to disasters. The MoFA harnesses contributions from humanitarian organizations to support the claim that Taiwan does a lot for people affected by crises, while arguing it could do more if offered observer status at the World Health Assembly.

Civil society organizations also interacted with the government in the WHO campaign through funding arrangements. The involvement of Rotary International is an interesting example. The ROC donated US$9.2 million to the WHO's polio eradication initiative (Taiwan Government Information Office, 2004). However, given political sensitivities, the donation was channelled through Rotary International. More precisely, the government donated $2 million while the public contributed the rest (e-mail from Benjamin Liu, 11 October 2004). Interestingly, in 2001 Taiwanese Gary Chi-Kuang Huang was elected vice-president of Rotary International (Rotary International, 2001).

Overseas, the FAPA promoted legislation in support of Taiwan's WHO bid. In addition, a number of associations, foundations and think tanks, in particular in North America and Europe, support Taiwan's WHO bid. Most importantly, large international medical associations in official relations with the WHO, including the World Medical Association (WMA), the International Pharmaceutical Federation (IPF), the International Council of Nursing (ICN) and the International Paediatrics Association (IPA), have supported Taiwan's WHO bid through press releases and occasionally in other ways. As an example,

> The International Council of Nurses (ICN), one of the three largest non-governmental international health organizations in the world, will host its 23rd Quadrennial Congress in Taipei from May 21–27. The conference is expected to draw more than 5,000 delegates from all over the world, an ICN spokesperson said in Geneva on Saturday. The congress, the biggest one hosted by an international non-governmental organization in Taiwan in recent years, will take place shortly after the World Health Assembly (WHA), which will run from May 16–25 in Geneva.
>
> (*Taipei Times*, 14 February 2005)

Governance outputs and outcomes: the WHO and Taiwan's bid for observer status

WHO: outputs and outcomes

Quantifying the WHO's output is difficult. Half of the funds the organization spends on programmes are allocated to six areas: immunization and vaccine development; HIV/AIDS; communicable disease prevention and control; malaria; tuberculosis; epidemic alert and response (WHO, 2004b). In contrast with other agencies, the WHO's output has more to do with expertise than funding for health services, like the World Bank, or delivery of physical inputs such as vaccines and drugs, like UNICEF.

The WHO's expertise in public health policy, technical advice or epidemiological surveillance is accessed through numerous publications including the *Bulletin of the World Health Organisation*, the *Weekly Epidemiological Record*, the *World Health Report* or other regional or thematic publications. Most of the expertise is not produced physically in WHO offices or laboratories but in hundreds of locations and institutions worldwide and an important part of the WHO's output is to link them up.

While the WHO is a recognized producer of numerous norms, standards and guidelines, the organization leaves frontline roles to others. The organization does not seek to match the Red Cross in emergency interventions, nor UNICEF in immunization logistics. In recent years, though, the WHO raised its operational profile as a frontline 'conductor' against emerging infectious diseases (Ebola, SARS, Marburg). The WHO also focuses on the next flu pandemic, which the organization says is inevitable.

One difficulty in evaluating the WHO's contribution is that national health authorities bear the primary responsibility for outputs and outcomes. In addition, other global organizations are involved in public health, including the World Bank, UNICEF, the UNAIDS and the Global Fund. Civil society organizations contribute significantly too, in particular as providers of health services to underprivileged sections of society.

Another difficulty results from the nature of part of the WHO's activities. Assessing the outcome of epidemiological surveillance is more difficult than measuring the impact of tobacco control measures. Should the WHO be praised if no flu pandemic occurs in the next ten or 20 years or could this be the 'lucky' consequence of viruses' low mutating abilities or other factors yet to be ascertained? Or, as suggested by a senior WHO official speculating on the range of casualties to be expected, should the outcome be regarded as positive if the number of deaths resulting from a flu pandemic is closer to five million than to 150 million? (*abcNews*, 30 September 2005).

The outputs and outcomes of Taiwan's campaign

Quantifying the output of Taiwan's WHO campaign is equally challenging. First, Taiwan's arguments in support of its bid are found in a variety of publications, including government websites, press and media, the websites of like-minded Taiwanese foundations, NGOs and other civil society organizations, and academic journals. They also appear in friendly publications overseas, electronic or in print, in parliamentary debates on both sides of the Atlantic and in pamphlets and leaflets distributed during demonstrations by Taiwanese activists in Geneva. Finally, they are invoked in the official requests that Taiwan's official diplomatic allies submit every year for inclusion in the agenda of the World Health Assembly.

The campaign is quite decentralized. New NGOs are created every year. The group at the origin of the campaign, the Foundation of Medical Professionals Association, split up into several organizations, which thereafter accorded various degrees of priority to the campaign.

Equally difficult to quantify is the cost of the campaign to Taiwanese taxpayers. The budget of the Ministry of Foreign Affairs lacks transparency. Besides, the diplomats involved in the WHO campaign also work on the UN campaign and similar political and humanitarian arguments are used for both campaigns.

Lastly, there is some ambiguity with regard to the intended outcome of the campaign. Interestingly, the executive summary of a concept paper is titled *Rebuttal to PRC arguments against inviting Taiwan as an observer of the WHA*, while the paper itself is titled *Rebuttal to PRC arguments against inviting Taiwan to participate in the WHO* (Taiwan Ministry of Foreign Affairs, undated). Does observership at the WHA equate participation in the WHO? In the absence of specific provisions for observer status in the WHO Constitution, the concept paper mentions the WHO's practice of allowing 'a number of "entities" to participate in the sessions of the World Health Assembly (WHA) as observers' (Taiwan Ministry of Foreign Affairs, undated: 4).

As each World Health Assembly is sovereign, observer status may be granted once and denied the following year. The concept paper anticipates this limitation and argues that the WHO's practice 'is well established and has given rise to *a new category of "quasi-permanent observers"* invited on a routine basis to the Assembly' (Taiwan Ministry of Foreign Affairs, undated: 4). The paper lists six such entities and concludes that 'these examples constitute powerful precedents for Taiwan's participation as an observer in the WHO' (Taiwan Ministry of Foreign Affairs, undated: 4), but Taiwan's bid will likely remain more controversial than the participation of the Vatican, the Red Cross or the Order of Malta. Taiwan's overriding objective may simply be to keep the Taiwan issue alive in international fora, an issue which is returned to in the next chapter.

Taiwan's campaign also produced unintended outcomes. Many delegates were unhappy with the lengthy discussion and vote at the 2004 Health Assembly. Some blamed Taiwan's friends and supporters, others China. Ahead of the fifty-eighth World Health Assembly, China floated the idea that Taiwanese experts might participate, as part of the Chinese delegation, in the WHO's technical work. 'State Councillor Tang Jiaxuan told a visiting delegation led by Chiang Pin-kung, the vice-chairman of Taiwan's opposition Kuomintang, in Beijing that the mainland had taken note of the Taiwanese public's desire to be part of the global health body' (*South China Morning Post*, 2 April 2005).

Taiwan's Premier Frank Hsieh later rejected a reported proposal to participate under the name 'Taiwan, China' as 'no more than a ploy to block Taiwan's participation in the World Health Organisation' (*China News Agency*, 4 April 2005). China signed a secret MoU with the WHO on 14 May 2005, the content of which was disclosed two weeks later by a KMT spokesman:

> 1. The WHO Secretariat can invite Taiwan's medical and public health experts to individually attend its technical activities. If necessary, Taiwan's experts can say they come from 'Taiwan, China.'
> 2. The WHO Secretariat can send its staff and experts to Taiwan to examine the public health and contagious disease situation as well as to discuss relevant health issues with Taiwan medical and public health experts and to provide medical and public health technical assistance to the island.
> 3. If Taiwan faces an outbreak of serious public health problems, the WHO Secretariat will, if necessary, send experts to Taiwan as soon as possible and give technical assistance to the island or invite Taiwan's medical and public health experts to join relevant technical activities initiated by the secretariat.
>
> (*Central News Agency*, 29 May 2005)

Taiwan's health minister protested against this agreement, seen as downgrading the island's status, and later on even stated that the agreement 'seriously hampers disease prevention efforts' (*Korea Times*, 4 April 2008). This important outcome was not the one Taiwan targeted, but Chen Shui-bian nonetheless acknowledged during a video-conference that

> In order to participate in the WHO or become an observer of the WHA, we have been working very hard in the last ten years. In the first eight years, we were not able to participate in any WHO-related technical meetings. But, in the last two years, we have been able to participate in 14 technical meetings.
>
> (Office of the President, Republic of China (Taiwan), 2006)

Another unintended outcome of Taiwan's bid is its impact on the WHO's NGO policy, as mentioned earlier. The mere suggestion that Taiwan might apply as an NGO was the most likely factor that pushed China to submit hastily drafted counterproposals. This eventually resulted in blocking the WHO's efforts to clarify and update its NGO policy.

Concluding comments and questions

Taiwan's bid is unusual in the history of the WHO. Taiwan says it is the victim of unique historical circumstances and portrays itself as both victim and rescuer in medical and humanitarian terms. The norms Taiwan refers to and the processes involved are therefore more complex than in the case of territorially-based applicants seeking to redress injustice resulting from colonial oppression. As these norms and processes have been examined in this chapter, it is now important to understand the unique characteristics of Taiwan's efforts to become an observer at the World Health Assembly. Why was this objective selected? How does it differ from any other bid? Does Taiwan comply with the norms it invokes? Are the actors involved working in unison? How does the Taiwan government link with organizations that support the bid at home and overseas? Are the policy instruments it uses appropriate? Is Taiwan likely to join the WHO? These questions are now addressed in the following chapter.

5 Taiwan's WHO campaign

Discussion

Introduction

Several sets of issues arising from the data provided in Chapter 4 are discussed here. The first set of issues relates to the governance norms Taiwan articulates in its WHO campaign. Are Taiwan's arguments relevant and credible? Are they consistent with the political, medical and humanitarian norms Taiwan invokes? How are political, humanitarian and medical arguments combined?

The second set of issues relates to governance actors. What can be learnt from this campaign with regard to the nature of the actors and organizations involved? Can these actors be clearly categorized? Is the division clear-cut between state and non-state organizations? Does the campaign help ascertain the nature of Taiwan?

A third set of issues relates to governance processes. How do the actors and organizations involved in Taiwan's campaign interact? How closely is Taiwan's bid linked with WHO governance processes in general? How effectively do Taiwanese authorities use the policy instruments at their disposal? Does its unclear status lead Taiwan to use atypical governance processes, i.e. processes not used by other entities seeking observer status at the WHO?

A fourth set of issues relates to governance ouputs and outcomes. Is it possible to better apprehend Taiwan's objective? Is Taiwan's strategy effective? Is Taiwan likely to join the WHO if it follows this strategy? Are there alternatives? Possible outcomes, intended or unintended, are then examined.

Governance norms revisited

Political norms

Taiwan focuses on three main political norms: universality, sovereignty and human rights. Taiwan says the current situation is a breach of the principle of universality at the core of the United Nations. How far does the WHO fail on this count? The question of the representation of China in the UN system arose after 1949. As countries from Eastern Europe withdrew from the WHO in 1949 and 1950, the PRC had very few diplomatic allies in the organization initially.

The PRC remained excluded from the UN and its specialized agencies for more than two decades, a numerically more significant breach of the principle of universality than the current exclusion of Taiwan: throughout the period, the PRC accounted for around one-fifth of the world population.

Communist regimes in divided states were also excluded during the same period, in particular North Korea, East Germany and North Vietnam. As Taiwan notes, East and West Germany were admitted as UN members simultaneously in 1973. North and South Korea were also admitted simultaneously in the UN in 1991. North Vietnam was admitted in 1975 and both halves of Vietnam united. But Taiwan never mentions that the Federal Republic of Germany became a WHO member in 1951, while the German Democratic Republic had to wait until 1973. Similarly, the Republic of Korea joined the WHO in 1948, whereas the Democratic Peoples' Republic of Korea was not admitted until 1991. Yemen, another divided country, also received differential treatment from the WHO. While Taiwan emphasizes that states representing divided nations were simultaneously admitted as UN members, Taiwan fails to acknowledge that this was not the case with the WHO.

More recently, the US forced the WHO to reject Palestine's membership application and threatened to stop funding any UN agency that would admit Palestine. The threat was significant, as the US is the top financial contributor to UN agencies, usually covering around one-quarter of their core budget. Agencies that lost US support and funding, such as UNESCO, were seriously affected.

True, the politics of exclusion also targeted anti-Communist regimes, such as Franco's Spain and South Africa's apartheid regime. The Spanish question, though, led to the establishment of voting rules more conducive to universal representation. The Soviet Union argued at the time that there should be a two-thirds majority to approve new members. This would have blocked Spain's bid, but instead a simple majority rule was established and Spain joined the WHO. After South Africa officially established apartheid in 1964, the World Health Assembly suspended the country's voting rights and privileges. South Africa withdrew from the WHO and was fully reinstated in 1994 after the apartheid regime collapsed.

The WHO is now more universal now than ever before, in particular during the first three decades of its existence, assuming the percentage of the world population represented in the organization is a relevant indicator. However, no Communist country was expelled from the WHO. Several withdrew at the beginning of the Cold War and did not seek readmission until 1956. Besides, the case of East Germany was not phrased in terms of exclusion, but in terms of 'deferred inclusion'. Taiwan is an exception. The issue, though, was not defined as the expulsion of a state but as the legitimate representation of China in the United Nations. In the 1950s and 1960s, the ROC never sought to include compatriots in the UN or the WHO. Nor did the Republic of China worry about the lack of representation for other Communist states seeking to represent divided nations such as Germany and Korea.

With regard to the sovereignty issue, Taiwan fulfils most of the criteria for statehood but lacks international recognition. Taiwan still enjoys the support of

23 UN members. Taken together, these countries only represent a tiny fraction of the world territory, population and GDP. Competition from China has reduced Taiwan's pool of diplomatic allies from 29 to 23 since 2000.

Taiwan refers to health rights as human rights: 'health for all' and access to healthcare, an issue which is addressed below. But human rights do not exist in a vacuum: the Universal Declaration of Human Rights and the United Nations Charter highlight the role of states as providers and guarantors of human rights. What would happen to the human rights currently enjoyed by Taiwanese if Taiwan were to be taken over by China? China mentioned that under the one-country, two-systems formula, Taiwan could keep its own system (democracy, rule of law), including its own armed forces. The PRC therefore claims, arguably, that Taiwanese compatriots should not fear that their own democratic system and human rights would be jeopardized. One obvious reason why they would is that, under Chinese pressure, the UN has barred Taiwanese journalists and media from covering the World Health Assembly since 2004. Reporters without Borders noted that this violates 'the Universal Declaration of Human Rights, article 19 of which guarantees press freedom and the free flow of information' and added that

> World Health Organisation director-general Margaret Chan rightly said at the opening of the World Health Assembly on 19 May 2008 that, 'Good health is a foundation for prosperity and contributes to stability, and these are assets in every country.' Except for Taiwan, one is tempted to add. Dr Chan called for 'balance in matters of health.' We call for balance in matters of news and information.
>
> (Reporters without Borders, 22 May 2008)

Lastly, one of Taiwan's political arguments, though historical and of lesser importance, should be put in perspective. The Republic of China claims that it was an active participant in the World Health Organization from 1948 to its expulsion in 1972, but official records do not speak in its favour. In particular, the Republic of China, though a founding member of the United Nations, withdrew from the WHO in 1950. The Republic of China returned to active participation in the organization three years later. From 1948 to 1972, the Republic of China sat only once on the Executive Board of the WHO. This is in stark contrast with the other permanent members of the UN Security Council. During the same period, the USSR sat 14 times on the Executive Board, the USA 19 times, the United Kingdom and France 20 times each. It is difficult to argue that the Republic of China's participation in the World Health Organization matched its rank. In contrast, this suggests that the Republic of China was not quite the active participant it now claims it was.

Scientific/medical/technical norms

Taiwanese officials argue that 'because of this exclusion, Taiwan cannot develop adequate health-care policies and is in no position to learn the latest international advances in medical science' (Tsai, 1999: 2157). There is an apparent contradiction between Taiwan's supposed inability to develop adequate healthcare policies and other facts mentioned in the same article:

> In the past few decades the ROC has accomplished considerable achievements in health. It enjoys one of the highest life expectancy levels in Asia, maternal and infant mortality rates are comparable with those of developed countries, it has eradicated infectious diseases such as malaria, smallpox, plague, and poliomyelitis, and it is the first country in the world to provide children with free hepatitis B vaccinations.
>
> (Tsai, 1999: 2157)

Are the author's assertions valid? The WHO does not provide data for Taiwan, but the CIA World Factbook estimated that in 2006 life expectancy in Taiwan was 77.43 years (74.67 years for males and 80.47 years for females) (Central Intelligence Agency, 2006a). This means that life expectancy in Taiwan is higher than in four out of five UN members and in particular higher than in Britain, Germany or the United States.

The author's claim is equally true with regard to infant mortality and maternal mortality. Taiwan has one of the lowest infant mortality and maternal mortality rates of all countries, as only 6.29 deaths are recorded for 1,000 live births (6.97 deaths/1,000 live births for males and 5.55 deaths/1,000 live births for females) (Central Intelligence Agency, 2006a). Taiwan has a lower infant mortality rate than the United States and most EU countries. In Asia, the only countries and territories where the infant mortality rate is lower than in Taiwan are Japan, Singapore, Hong Kong and Macao. In fact, infant mortality is lower in Taiwan than in more than 90 per cent of WHO member countries. This is a remarkable achievement.

One should certainly look at these data critically. What matters here is not so much a snapshot of current public health data as the cumulative impact, if any, of Taiwan's exclusion from the WHO over time on its ability to enhance public health. There again, Taiwan's argument that its exclusion from the WHO hampered its capacity to devise effective public health strategies does not stand scrutiny. During the 1972–2005 period, life expectancy rose from 67.6 years to 74.67 years for men and from 72.3 to 80.47 years for women. Taiwan progressed significantly outside the WHO, at a pace comparable to other developed economies. Taiwan's health authorities and the Centre of Disease Control recognize that the determinants of the health status of a population are manifold. In particular, as the level of economic development rises, the level of education also rises, and so does the proportion of a country's wealth devoted to healthcare.

Could observer status help Taiwan to do even better in terms of public health? Would Taiwan learn anything it does not already know? Ironically, the top two performers in terms of life expectancy and infant mortality are Andorra and Macao, two territories loosely connected with the WHO. Andorra joined only in 1997. The Macao SAR is neither a WHO member nor an associate member. It is not even an observer. This undermines Taiwan's argument that joining the WHO would lead to improved health outcomes.

As the World Health Assembly is more a political decision-making body than a forum where critical or cutting-edge medical information is shared, Taiwan's claim that it 'cannot develop adequate health-care policies and is in no position to learn the latest international advances in medical science' remains unsubstantiated (Tsai, 1999: 2157).

What impact would observer status have on Taiwan's ability to share its medical expertise globally and improve global health outcomes? There are simply too many variables to consider. Medical research is primarily disseminated through hundreds of medical journals around the world. Reading them does not require any connection with the WHO. Access to search engines such as Medline and databases such as ProMED, which tracks outbreaks of infectious diseases around the world, is not restricted to WHO members.

In addition, the argument that Taiwan could and would do more in terms of sharing medical knowledge and research if it were made an observer at the World Health Assembly is a double-edged sword. Taiwan's authorities certainly do not suggest that they could refrain from sharing important medical information because they do not have observer status with the WHO.

Humanitarian norms

While epidemic outbreaks involve the WHO's core expertise, the WHO's role in response to natural disasters is marginal. The WHO does not have the operational or logistical capacity to immunize or treat patients in case of a large-scale outbreak in a resource-poor country. This is primarily the responsibility of national health authorities. Where needed, UNICEF and specialized medical international NGOs such as MSF are ready to step in.

Local hospitals are the frontline responders to epidemic outbreaks in resource-rich countries such as Taiwan. They are usually linked up in a comprehensive, nationwide epidemiological surveillance and alert network. There is no need for UNICEF or other UN operational agencies to intervene. The WHO's expertise primarily relies on the input of relevant agencies in resource-rich countries. The range of communicable diseases prevalent in such countries is also much narrower than in less developed countries. In Taiwan,

> Plague and smallpox have long been eradicated. No cases of rabies have been reported since 1959. Malaria was declared eradicated by the WHO in 1965. Other communicable diseases such as diphtheria, pertussis, tetanus, polio, Japanese encephalitis, and tuberculosis are under effective control. No confirmed polio cases of wild strain have been reported since 1984.
>
> (Chan, 1998)

The epidemic outbreaks Taiwan refers to in its WHO campaign must be assessed against this background. The low number of fatal cases is a reflection on the effectiveness of the systems of epidemiological surveillance and response to outbreaks in developed countries.

Although the epidemiology of cancer, cardiovascular diseases or obesity is more relevant to the health status of populations in developed countries, epidemic outbreaks of contagious diseases still have a strong emotional impact. Even minor outbreaks of infectious diseases in the developed world receive a disproportionate level of attention.

In the case of the enterovirus 71 outbreak in 1998, Taiwan claims that 'the PRC prevented WHO experts from helping Taiwan combat a deadly outbreak of enterovirus' (Taiwan Ministry of Foreign Affairs, undated: 7), while acknowledging that 'foreign assistance did come, but only belatedly and indirectly through private channels' (Gao, 2004). These channels, though, were not private:

> The experts, who arrived Saturday from the U.S. Centers for Disease Control and Prevention in Atlanta, are to stay in Taiwan for up to four weeks to investigate the virus, which has also been detected in Bulgaria and in Malaysia where an outbreak last year killed 30 children. 'It looks like these children had got brain infections and died suddenly,' said U.S. epidemic intelligence officer Anthony Mounts, referring to the deaths in Taiwan. 'They died so swiftly and ... because of the lack of autopsy ... it's very difficult to know whether they died of the virus.' The U.S. scientists also were meeting with Taiwanese health officials to discuss 'preventive measures,' Hsu said.
>
> (*CNN.com*, 8 June 1998)

On its Communicable Disease Surveillance and Response website the WHO reported that 'local health authorities and a team from the Centers for Disease Control and Prevention in Atlanta, USA, continue to investigate the outbreak' (WHO, 1998b). Although it is not clear whether Taiwan requested help from the WHO, whether the WHO forwarded the request to the US CDC, or whether China blocked the WHO from doing anything, it is clear that Taiwan received support not from a 'private' source, but from the most relevant and competent agency of the US government. Taiwan nonetheless claimed that it was abandoned by the international medical community.

It is also doubtful whether observer status at the World Health Assembly would have made any difference. Taiwan's health authorities complained that they did not get adequate information on the 1997 enterovirus 71 outbreak in Malaysia (Chan *et al.*, 2000), which they argue could have helped them tackle the outbreak in Taiwan. True, researchers writing on the 1997 episode in Malaysia noted similarities between the two outbreaks, but they also pointed to a number of unresolved questions and uncertainties with regard to the aetiology of the disease and the number of agents that might have been involved (Chan *et al.*, 2000).

The lack of information does not appear to have been intentional. The WHO may not have established clear case definition and treatment guidelines when the outbreak occurred. The WHO's Global Outbreak Alert and Response Network was still fledgling and not fully operational. In addition, member states are not always forthcoming when it comes to reporting epidemic outbreaks, as was initially the case for China with regard to SARS, and as might have been the case with Malaysia at the time. Indeed, the role of the WHO is to disseminate the information reported by member states, but the organization does not have the power to investigate in the absence of a member state's request and authorization.

Undoubtedly, some of China's actions in the case of the Chi-Chi earthquake were not understood by the international community and led to a legitimate uproar in Taiwan. In particular, barring a Russian plane carrying aid from its airspace was counterproductive if China wanted to convince global public opinion that it cared for Taiwanese people. Everyone is aware that China has a weak public health infrastructure and cannot provide decent healthcare to many of its citizens. Most developing countries understand this, as they face similar problems. But one thing is for China to rhetorically assert that it takes charge of the health of Taiwanese compatriots when everyone knows it cannot. Another thing is to use physical instruments, such as flight restrictions, to delay the arrival of aid or insist that countries willing to assist Taiwan first ask for Beijing's authorization.

Unlike UNICEF, the WHO has only a marginal role in response to natural disasters. Delays in assisting Taiwan after the Chi-Chi earthquake had nothing to do with Taiwan's exclusion from the WHO but resulted from China's obstruction. The UNOCHA plays an important role in despatching information through its website, Reliefweb, used by UN agencies and NGOs alike. The Taiwanese government complained that a UNOCHA fact-finding mission was delayed under pressure from Beijing, but Reliefweb posted messages and updates sent by every agency involved.

Many governments responded to Taiwan's appeals. Interestingly, professional rescue teams with sniffer dogs and specialized equipment were sent by the governments of many countries and territories which do not officially recognize Taiwan, including Japan, Singapore, Hong Kong, Mexico, the United States, France and Germany. This surprised many in Taiwan, and had several consequences.

The efficiency of foreign rescue teams contrasted the disorganization of official relief efforts. The media and NGOs like Tzu Chi criticized the government's slow response. In some instances foreign rescue teams were kept idle or directed to locations where other rescue teams had already been despatched. The whole episode was an embarrassment for the government and exposed serious deficiencies in crisis response. Blaming China's pressure and attempts to delay international relief efforts may therefore have been in part an attempt to deflect criticism. There was no demonstrable link, however indirect, between the suffering of Taiwanese people and the WHO. Had Taiwan been an observer at the time, it would not have made any difference. The WHO simply does not have the operational capacity to respond to such disasters. The WHO's response was in the form of a cash grant from its Department of Emergency and Humanitarian Action, as is the case in similar circumstances. The US$50,000 grant was channelled through the International Federation of the Red Cross and Red Crescent Societies, which forwarded it to the Taiwanese Red Cross. The Federation acknowledged receipt by fax dated 6 November 1999. WHO informed the Ministry of Health of the PRC and the Permanent Representative of China to the United Nations in Geneva of the grant and its purpose by letter of 6 June 2000.

In the case of the SARS episode in 2003, Taiwan also made unfounded claims. WHO officials were unhappy with Taiwan's claim that the WHO ignored requests for help. To counter this widely publicized claim, they took the unusual step to write a summary of events (WHO, 2003c) detailing the WHO's response to requests from Taiwan.

The WHO first pointed out that through its Global Outbreak Alert and Response Network, it seeks to promote the 'prompt exchange of relevant information concerning disease outbreaks [including] epidemiological information, case identification, treatment and recommended public health measures [and] when appropriate, field visits by either WHO itself or other centres collaborating with it' (WHO, 2003c: 1). In response to SARS specifically, the document stated, 'WHO and its partner institutes and collaborating centres have placed field teams in China; the Hong Kong Special Administrative Region of China; Taiwan, China; and Vietnam' (WHO, 2003c: 1).

On 14 March, the WHO was notified of two suspect cases of atypical pneumonia by the Director-General of Taiwan's Center for Disease Control. The message

> was promptly transmitted by WHO, as in the case of other notifications, to the appropriate WHO Collaborating Centre: in this case the Centers for Disease Control and Prevention (CDC) in Atlanta, which also has a field centre in Taiwan, China. The notification was accompanied by a request for CDC follow-up assistance in the field. CDC Atlanta swiftly acknowledged the request and agreed to follow-up. A further request for advice from Taiwan, China sent to WHO Geneva and WHO Manila was received later in the day.
>
> (WHO, 2003c: 1)

On 16 March, 'two CDC staff members arrived in Taipei from Thailand'. Authorities in Taiwan complained that they had not received any response from the WHO, but the WHO confirmed that 'the initial request had indeed been passed to CDC Atlanta as soon as it had been received'. To further clarify the point, on 20 March,

> a fax was sent by Dr Guénaël Rodier, Director, Communicable Disease Surveillance and Response Department, WHO, Geneva to Dr Chen acknowledging the messages of 14 and 15 March, and reiterating the point made by the WHO Executive Director of Communicable Diseases on Sunday, confirming that CDC Atlanta had been contacted.
>
> (WHO, 2003c: 2)

Finally the next day, 'an e-mail acknowledgement was sent from WHO Geneva to CDC DoH Taiwan, China with respect to information sent to date on cases of

SARS and their investigation' (WHO, 2003c: 2). It is therefore remarkable that Taiwan complained at the time, and even more remarkable that Taiwan still complains, that the 'WHO did not respond for almost 7 weeks to the request for help from Taiwan' (Taiwan Ministry of Foreign Affairs, 2005a: 6). Obviously, health authorities in Taiwan must be aware that in order to respond to epidemic outbreaks the WHO mobilizes its network of collaborating centres. No less obviously, they must be familiar with the US Centre of Disease Control, which has a field centre in Taiwan and helped Taiwan at the time of the enterovirus 71 in 1998. So the only plausible explanation for Taiwan's persistence in denying that the WHO responded to their request is complete formalism, i.e. they did not regard the sending of a CDC team as a response from the WHO, although the WHO confirmed it had requested the US CDC to assist. This is clearly a victory of form over substance.

There was an upsurge of the epidemic at the end of April and in particular an acceleration of hospital infections as mentioned earlier. On 3 May, in response to this unfortunate development, 'a two-person WHO team with expertise in epidemiology and virology arrived in Taipei, Taiwan, China to support health authorities in combating the SARS outbreak' (WHO, 2003c: 3). On 16 May, two public health experts from Taiwan participated in a WHO consultation on SARS and in late June, experts from Taiwan participated in a regional conference on SARS in Bangkok.

On one occasion, though, Taiwan's hopes to participate were dashed. This was during a technical briefing of the World Health Assembly. Newly appointed Minister of Health Chen Chien-jen flew to Geneva hoping he would be allowed to speak about Taiwan's fight against SARS. Although the briefing was labelled as 'technical', the fact that it was held as part of the World Health Assembly led to high hopes and expectations in the Taiwanese press:

> It would be the first time that a Taiwanese official has been invited to speak on a WHO-held occasion since the nation was excluded from the world health body in 1972. … Chen is scheduled to present a three-minute report on the development of SARS in Taiwan during the WHA technical briefing. If he is allowed a chance to speak, Chen will be the first Taiwanese official to attend a WHA meeting for 30 years.
>
> (*Taipei Times*, 19 May 2003b)

Taiwan was eventually barred from making a presentation during the briefing. Taiwan's Minister of Health apparently had mixed feelings about being shut out. He insisted that the purpose was to share Taiwan's experience in handling SARS, which he felt was a technical issue, not a political one. But he recognized that Taiwan was maybe too naïve to think that his participation would not be affected by politics. He also acknowledged the value of an earlier teleconference organized by Dr David Heymann, then Executive Director of Communicable Diseases at the WHO. In contrast, Taiwan's Minister of Foreign Affairs Eugene Chien was highly critical of China's attitude:

> 'The Chinese government should apologize to the people of Taiwan for having hurt the hearts of the 23 million people here by obstructing our bid to join the international health system,' Chien said yesterday … 'It's a question of humanitarian concerns, a question about lives and deaths. It's not a move to create "one China, one Taiwan" or about splitting China. Such an argument can only hurt the feelings of the Taiwanese people,' Chien said. Beijing's attempts to belittle Taiwan in the international community were detrimental to cross-strait relations, Chien said.
>
> (*Taipei Times*, 21 May 2003)

Overall, Taiwan's claim that it suffered because of its exclusion from the WHO is again misplaced in the case of SARS. Taiwan suffered, like other countries and territories, from China's initial cover-up of the epidemic. In terms of morbidity, Taiwan was considerably less affected than Hong Kong, but the case fatality rate was comparable (20 per cent in Taiwan, 17 per cent in Hong Kong). The difference is that Hong Kong took decisive action, in spite of initial blunders, and focused its energy on fighting the disease head-on. Most noticeable was the selfless attitude of frontline medical workers. Besides, Hong Kong was at the forefront of research efforts to identify the cause of the epidemic. In contrast, Taiwan spent a lot of energy on formal controversies and the government tried to capitalize on the whole episode to achieve diplomatic gains at the World Health Assembly.

Evidence is weak that Taiwan's suffering could have been reduced during any of the three emergencies, had the island been an observer at the World Health Assembly. The issue of Taiwan's aid to countries affected by man-made or natural disasters is addressed later. Could Taiwan do more, or better, if granted observer status at the World Health Assembly? This and other issues relevant to Taiwan's aid programmes are discussed in Chapters 6 and 7.

Norms combined

How effectively does the combination of political and humanitarian arguments and norms help build Taiwan's case for WHO observership? Taiwan insists that it is only concerned with the health of human beings in Taiwan and elsewhere. But the common thread between the three emergencies discussed here is not the WHO, it is China's interference. Specifically, Taiwan accuses the PRC of refusing to acknowledge the nature of its request: Taiwan does not apply for membership, although it says it meets the criteria for statehood, and emphasizes that UN membership is not a prerequisite for WHO membership. For instance, from 1946 to 2000, Switzerland was a WHO member but not a UN member. Similarly, Niue and the Cook Islands are WHO members but not UN members. Instead, Taiwan insists that its application for observer status does not interfere with China's claim of sovereignty over Taiwan.

When a disaster strikes Taiwan, China is invariably accused of 'politicizing' the issue, i.e. trying to extract some political advantage from the suffering of the

Taiwanese people. In 1998, Taiwan accused China of preventing the WHO from helping Taiwan fight the enterovirus 71 outbreak. In 1999, Taiwan complained about flight restrictions and China's insistence that offers of help had to be cleared by authorities in Beijing. In 2003, Taiwan accused China of blocking WHO experts from coming to Taiwan to assist in efforts to contain SARS.

'Politicization' works both ways. The PRC says that, whenever disaster strikes, the Taiwanese authorities try to gain some political advantage, call for interference in China's internal affairs and take small steps towards independence. In particular, exchanges between both sides of the strait after the Chi-Chi earthquake highlighted a complex pattern. Initially, Taiwan's authorities 'expressed appreciation to the mainland Chinese authorities for their offer of assistance and relief funds' (*Taiwan News*, 23 September 1999a), but immediately added that they 'needed to deliberate further before deciding whether to accept their offer' (*Taiwan News*, 23 September 1999a).

The deputy secretary-general of the Strait Exchange Foundation said 'help would be welcomed as long as cross-strait politics stayed out of the way' but emphasized that 'rescuers or relief workers from the mainland would have to … demonstrate that they had no political motives, something that is not asked of teams from other countries' (*Taiwan News*, 23 September 1999a). This certainly indicates how difficult it is to keep politics out of cross-strait disaster relief.

In addition, and in response to an offer of aid by the Chinese Red Cross, an official of the Taiwanese Red Cross said: 'We don't have special needs for a Red Cross team from China to come now' (*Taiwan News*, 23 September 1999b). Taiwanese officials also criticized the Chinese Red Cross for demanding that 'its counterparts in other countries around the world should seek mainland approval before offering aid to Taiwan's quake victims' (*China News Agency*, 23 September 1999). Another Taiwanese official criticized the PRC for thanking foreign countries that offered humanitarian aid to the people of Taiwan and added that 'Taiwan had never raised any political terms while offering humanitarian aid to mainland compatriots suffering from national disasters' (*Taiwan News*, 23 September 1999a). The problem is that such a statement about aid is also highly political.

Humanitarian arguments are necessarily ambivalent when used by states, as they are powerful symbolic policy instruments. They illustrate links between norms and instruments, as no state can prove that it is disinterested when it uses such arguments. It is always possible to show how a state benefits politically from using a given humanitarian argument. When China says, as it did during the SARS episode in 2003, that it helps Taiwan in many ways, China is obviously under pressure to show that it is doing something. The stakes were high in the run-up to the Health Assembly. China was widely criticized for its handling of the SARS outbreak and worried that Taiwan would receive increased support for its observer status bid. China therefore did not object to the visit of WHO-mandated experts to Taiwan in early May, ahead of the Health Assembly. China also agreed to Taiwanese participation in a SARS conference in Bangkok in June. When the WHO responded to Taiwan's request for help on 3 May, China went as far as saying that it had authorized the visit. In a very unusual twist, a WHO spokesman flatly denied that such authorization had been sought or given.

Taiwan says there are no ulterior, political motives to its application for observer status, but it is easy to find some. Observer status with the WHO has sometimes been described as a stepping-stone towards UN membership. Nothing in Taiwan's WHO campaign strategy suggests that medical needs or humanitarian imperatives are its only motives. There is little evidence of efforts by Taiwan to get involved in serious medical or epidemiological work with relevant WHO institutions, although the Taiwanese CDC applied to become part of the GOARN and its application was turned down. In a video-conference, Chen Shui-bian questioned the rationale behind Taiwan's exclusion and thanked Western countries for supporting Taiwan CDC's application to join the GOARN (Office of the President, Republic of China (Taiwan), 2006).

In the 1990s consultants hired by the government suggested alternative strategies. Taiwan, they advised, would gain respect and exposure by getting involved in substantive programmes, such as the Tropical Disease Research (TDR) programme located at WHO headquarters in Geneva and jointly run by the WHO, the UNDP and the World Bank. Neither the KMT nor the DPP showed interest in such a strategy. There is only limited evidence of Taiwan's interest or involvement in such groundwork, far from the spotlight, on medical and epidemiological issues. In the past few years research articles were published by Taiwanese medical teams in Malawi (see for example Yu *et al.*, 2005, 2007 and 2008) and São Tomé (Lien *et al.*, 2008). Taiwan's medical assistance to both countries is discussed in Chapters 6 and 7.

The WHO campaign relies primarily on lobbying, press and media work and high-profile activism at the time of the Health Assembly. Maybe Taiwanese officials do not think that substantive contributions and groundwork of little media value would make a difference anyway. Taiwan may reason that its emotional appeal to public opinion is more effective or that, regardless of arguments and contributions, WHO members vote according to their interests. If this is the case, Taiwan may regard low-key, measurable contributions towards the advancement of global health as irrelevant to its efforts to gain observer status.

Governance actors revisited

State actors

One of the main issues raised by the case study is the nature of Taiwan and its international status. In most respects, Taiwan behaves like a state but suffers from low external recognition and lack of domestic consensus on its identity. If Taiwan is not a sovereign entity, what is it? The concept of quasi-state was suggested in the case of Hong Kong, which has some measure of international recognition and responsibility for certain aspects of its international relations (Tang, 1993). These aspects, though, were not defined by Hong Kong but by Britain and China. China agreed to Taiwan's participation in some intergovernmental organizations, such as the ADB, APEC or the WTO, where membership is not restricted to sovereign states. China also agreed to Hong Kong's participation in the same organizations. The issue is: can Taiwan gain a foothold in any intergovernmental organization, even as a simple observer with no voting rights, against China's will?

Taiwan's participation in the WHO remains, at the time of writing, an unresolved issue. Taiwan might one day become an observer. Or it might apply as an NGO, as suggested by a delegate at the fifty-sixth Health Assembly. Or it might even one day, if recognized as a sovereign state, gain full membership. Or Taiwan could, if reunited with China, become an associate member. These various options are not just theoretical possibilities: they highlight the uncertain nature of some entities in the global arena. Palestine sought full membership, but was denied it and made an observer under US pressure. The Holy See could have applied for full membership, but chose instead to become an observer. The ICRC was an NGO in official relations with the WHO, but later on applied to be admitted as an observer after being invited as such by the UN. The IFRC followed suit. When the Sovereign Order of Malta applied to become an NGO in official relations, the WHO's Standing Committee deferred its response, as it could not ascertain the nature of the organization. The Sovereign Order of Malta was eventually made an observer.

In the main committees of the UN General Assembly, observers are usually

> given permission to 'address the organ' or 'to speak when invited' or to 'speak when invited by the Chairman'. Implementation depends to a large degree on the 'status' of the observer, the importance of the issue to the observer and the character of the meeting to be attended.
>
> (Sohn, 1996: 162)

But in granting observer status to Palestine, the fifty-third World Health Assembly referred to the modalities decided by the UN General Assembly, including the 'right of reply', 'the right to co-sponsor draft resolutions and decisions on Palestinian and Middle East issues' and 'the right to make interventions, with a precursory explanation or the recall of relevant General Assembly resolutions being made only once by the President of the General Assembly at the start of each session of the Assembly' (WHO, 2000a: 5).

The rights and obligations of observers are negotiable, if not tailor-made, as they were not clearly established when the WHO was set up. The case of Palestine also suggests that applications for the status of 'quasi-permanent observer' by territorial entities with problematic statehood claims will be handled by member states directly and not delegated to the Director-General (Sohn, 1996; Burci and Vignes, 2004). In addition,

> the granting of observer status to a 'controversial' entity may give rise to disputes and difficulties. The admittance of the PLO as an observer in the International Labour Organization, for example, caused the United States to withdraw from this organization.
>
> (Sybesma-Knol, 1996: 186)

This suggests that the status of some entities in the international arena is not predetermined, but results from interactions and mutual adjustments. What status does a given entity seek? What status is the international community ready to grant? Taiwan describes itself variously as a 'customs territory', as in the case of the WTO, an 'economy' in the case of APEC and a 'fishing entity' in several maritime treaties and organizations. These descriptions match the official terminology used for entities other than states in these organizations and agreements. But Taiwan breaks new ground when it applies as a 'health entity' to join the WHO as an observer, as there is no mention of such entities in WHO statutes.

Observer status appears to be a perfect decoy. At first sight it may appear as an innocuous outcome Taiwan says it seeks, but achieving observership may be just one step in a long process. Applying for observer status helps Taiwan keep the sovereignty issue alive and aside at the same time. To express this in the terms of the analytical framework used here, the outcome may turn out to be just a policy instrument in this case. How does the status of WHO observers evolve over time? Once observer status is granted to a given 'entity', there is no fixed or determined path for the future. An observer may remain an observer. The Holy See could in theory apply for membership, but may be satisfied to influence WHO policies, primarily in reproductive health, through other states, diplomatic envoys and the church structure (Mumford, 1992; Flanders, 1999; interview with a senior WHO executive, Geneva, 16 June 2003). The Sovereign Order of Malta has been an observer since 1963 and presumably does not plan to apply for membership, even though the Order has bilateral diplomatic relations with 100 countries (Sovereign Order of Malta, 2008). The ANC saw its observer status revoked by the World Health Assembly when the apartheid regime was abolished, the ANC became the ruling party of the newly democratic South Africa and the country's membership was restored.

An observer may also become a member, as was the case with the German Democratic Republic and others in the past, and could be the case for Palestine in the future. Taiwan seems to hint at this possibility when it recalls that the Republic of China was the only founder member of the United Nations to insist that territories under trusteeship [i.e. non-sovereign] be given over time the opportunity to move towards independence.

One interesting point is that entities can apply independently for three of the four statuses mentioned above: member, observer and NGO in official relations. The only status for which an entity cannot apply on its own is associate membership. In any case, when Taiwan insists that it is applying for observer status and not membership in order to put the sovereignty issue aside and focus on health matters exclusively, it certainly keeps open the possibility of moving towards UN membership via WHO membership. The World Health Assembly can accept states applying for membership by a simple majority vote

> This easy procedural requirement together with the absence of any possibility of a 'veto' as in the UN's Security Council, clearly reveals why WHO has been the first choice of these countries wishing to enter the UN family

> whose application might be considered controversial or whose international status might be uncertain.
>
> (Burci and Vignes, 2004: 22)

Besides, the Director-General appears to have more than a procedural role as it is not clear whether he or she has the responsibility to assess an applicant's credentials or must simply transmit to members 'any application sent by any entity claiming statehood' (Burci and Vignes, 2004: 23).

Indeed, Taiwan blew its cover in 2007 and 2008 when it applied for full membership under the name of Taiwan. The main reason stated for the change of tack was impatience, if not exasperation, with the lack of results from the bid for observer status. 'Most countries still reject outright our reasonable and moderate appeal. As a result, people in Taiwan are becoming impatient and expect the government to show its determination by adopting new approaches' (Taiwanese Young Professionals Association of Quebec, 2007). Taiwan therefore reframed the objective and acknowledged that observer status was a path to membership, noting that 'according to rule 3 of the WHA rules of procedure "the Director-General of the World Health Organization may invite States having made application for membership to send observers to sessions of the World Health Assembly"' (Taiwan Government, 2008: 2). It was also noted that a precedent existed, as 'East Germany was invited by the Director-General to become a WHA observer in 1972' (Taiwan Government, 2008: 2).

It is interesting that Taiwan refers to the German Democratic Republic precedent, as the case showed that the Director-General has some latitude in deciding whether or not to invite entities applying for membership to send observers to the Health Assembly (Burci and Vignes, 2004). The Director-General could invite Taiwan as an observer but is unlikely to do so in the absence of an overwhelming consensus among members. The election of Margaret Chan as Director-General makes it even less likely, unless of course China requests her to do so.

The WHO was described as an international organization paralyzed by divisions and conflicts between member states (Badie, 2002). The WHO does not seem to conform to the liberal view of international organizations as engines of global norm-setting but appears to be riddled with conflicts. The issue of Taiwan's representation in the WHO is a case in point but not the only one: the WHO's NGO policy, discussed in Chapter 4, is another example.

Besides, norm-setting at the WHO is affected by other state and non-state actors, including religious groups and multinational pharmaceutical companies. Another important institutional aspect is that the WHO lost or abandoned part of its mandate to other IGOs over time, such as the World Bank, UNAIDS, UNFPA or the Global Fund. This point is examined in Chapter 6.

Non-state actors

Some organizations, such as the Federation of Medical Professionals in Taiwan, are not easily categorized: the FMPAT appears to be involving both for-profit and non-profit organizations. The state encourages Taiwanese non-state organizations to play unofficial diplomatic roles. The KMT pushed the corporate sector to establish contacts with top foreign officials, while NGOs were generally seen as oppositional. The Chen Shui-bian administration tried to involve NGOs more systematically in diplomatic efforts. How far did it succeed? This issue is addressed in the following chapters.

China tried to counter Taiwan's numerous NGO initiatives but was less successful, as China's relationships with foreign NGOs have long been strained. China often views Western NGOs with suspicion, while many NGOs are critical of China's human rights record. In the case of medical NGOs, this is compounded by medical ethics concerns. Overall, China is in a defensive mode towards NGOs. In particular, China acts as a gatekeeper at the UN Standing Committee on NGOs, scrutinizes INGO applications for accreditation and assesses them on the basis of several criteria, including their positions on the Taiwan and Tibet issues.

Some Taiwanese NGOs openly or unofficially favour reunification. In a report the PRC mission to the UN in Geneva stated that 'the representative of the Taipei Medical Association has recently visited the mainland' on a SARS mission (Permanent Mission of the Peoples' Republic of China to the United Nations office at Geneva, 2003). But most Taiwanese medical NGOs support Taiwan's WHO campaign.

Governance processes revisited

The focus here is again on governance processes as defined in Chapter 2 in terms of linking arrangements and policy instruments. State-to-state interactions are discussed first before turning to civil society interactions. The combination of both types of processes is discussed thereafter.

State-to-state interactions

Though primarily shaped by state interests and the distribution of power, state-to-state interactions within WHO remain constrained by numerous rules. Procedural rules were selected to improve on earlier and less successful attempts at international health cooperation and enhance international cooperation through the United Nations. They define a framework through which states interact, but also through which the distribution of power can be assessed.

In 1971, Taiwan did not measure US support for its cause by what the US said. What Taiwan was interested to know was whether the US would invoke the 'important question' rule, as it had done so far with regard to the representation of China, and request a two-thirds majority instead of a simple one. The invocation of the 'important question' rule was thus a measure of the relative power of the US and the PRC at the time and of the relative importance of Taiwan's status for the US.

Similarly, Taiwan does not measure the progress of its cause by the quality of arguments deployed in World Health Assembly debates. The yardstick, instead, is the number and relative power of countries which support the inclusion of the question of Taiwan's representation in the agenda of the World Health Assembly. The extent of China's power is confirmed as this question was never included in the agenda of the World Health Assembly, even as a supplementary item. Conversely, Taiwan enjoys some measure of success when the Health Assembly is forced to debate and vote on the inclusion of the proposal in its agenda.

Civil society interactions

The civil society process in support of Taiwan's WHO bid is enthusiastic but appears to be so far limited in scope. Do Taiwanese NGOs really know how the WHO works? Are they aware of the great diversity of operational modes tested and implemented by thousands of NGOs around the world? This is an area for further research, as the case study suggests that Taiwanese medical NGOs have only explored a narrow range of possibilities and mainly focused on operational modes that directly target states and IGOs. Exceptions include those involved in overseas medical assistance programmes (see Chapter 6). The contribution of Taiwanese medical organizations is nonetheless remarkable as they managed to mobilize global medical associations over time and led them to re-express support for Taiwan's yearly bid at the Health Assembly. In particular, the WMA, IPF and ICN have formed an umbrella group, the World Health Professionals Alliance (WHPA), which supports Taiwan's WHO bid.

Overseas Taiwanese organizations also play a critical role. In particular, the FAPA has achieved impressive results with regard to Taiwan-related legislation in the US Congress. But it is not clear whether there is really a transnational process at work. Numerous civil society organizations support Taiwan, but they have not formed any kind of 'global alliance for Taiwan in the WHO'. Such an alliance may be formed in the future, but so far the various groups involved do not seem to collaborate closely. Geneva-based international NGOs primarily target the WHO and other IGOs. The FAPA focuses on the US public opinion and Congress. Taiwanese NGOs may be more closely related to domestic political debates. There is no clear evidence of a global civil society dynamic in this case.

State and non-state processes combined

States try to harness and control the power of non-state organizations. Some states, including China, firmly seek to control NGOs. The WHO tried to devise a policy towards market organizations and attempted to define what constitutes a conflict of interest, but the draft policy paper was never submitted to the Board or the Assembly. As discussed earlier, the US refused to distinguish market organizations from NGOs. This appears to strengthen the position of market organizations within the WHO. In particular, Western pharmaceutical companies have in many instances contracted with the WHO to set up programmes designed to fight infectious diseases, known as Global Public–Private Partnerships (GPPPs). These partnerships were found to have limited legitimacy (Buse and Walt, 2000). Besides, it is difficult to assess the costs and benefits of such programmes, either with regard to the production of global public goods or for pharmaceutical companies (Guilloux and Moon, 2000). One concern is the impact of GPPPs on the WHO's policy-making role: 'Will WHO maintain sufficient centrality to forge a coherent global agenda?' (Buse and Walt, 2000: 17).

The WHO recognizes that NGOs/CSOs contribute to policy-making and implementation and notes that they can 'bring up sensitive issues that WHO, as an intergovernmental organisation, may not be in a position to address for political reasons' (WHO, 2002c: 13). This is an indirect acknowledgement that WHO policy is not dictated by one type of actor alone, be they state, market or civil society forces, but results from the interaction of all these forces.

The WHO also acknowledges that cooperating with NGOs/CSOs enhances visibility and accountability, although the WHO does not have civil society representatives on its board, unlike the UNAIDS. WHO procedures only relate to those INGOs in official relations with the WHO at headquarter level. CSOs/NGOs at regional or country level are unclear about concrete possibilities of interaction with the WHO, while aid funds are increasingly channelled through these organizations.

Wary of NGO influence in the WHO as in the whole UN system, China watches very closely Taiwan's efforts to be readmitted in the United Nations. A five-member Standing Committee on NGOs scrutinizes the applications of INGOs seeking accreditation with the WHO. Wherever the applicant has a Taiwan chapter, China opposes any representation that refers to the 'Republic of China'. China screens in the same way NGOs seeking accreditation with the Economic and Social Council.

As China's vigilant monitoring of NGO accreditation policies in the UN system is well established, it does not seem to offer a convincing explanation of China's abrupt and radical change of attitude at the fifty-sixth World Health Assembly. China possibly worried about the weakening of its position following the SARS crisis, which was on everyone's mind at the time. China was criticized for its handling of the SARS episode and in particular for the cover-up of critical epidemiological information in the initial phase of the outbreak. Taiwan, in turn, was quick to seize the opportunity and tried to capitalize on this episode.

Taiwan's bid for observer status failed as usual on the first day of the Health Assembly. The most likely reason for China's change of mind therefore appears to be an impromptu declaration by an EU delegate during the Taiwan debate, who reportedly said that if Taiwan's application for observer status was rejected, the island could always re-apply as an NGO. Although there is no unquestionable evidence to support this analysis, several insiders think that this is what triggered China's change of mind and frantic redrafting of its proposal on the WHO's NGO policy (personal communications of WHO officers, Geneva, 16 and 18 June 2003). The Taiwan issue very likely had a major impact on global rules guiding the WHO's interactions with NGOs.

Governance outputs and outcomes revisited

Taiwan's outputs in perspective

How far do Taiwan's arguments reach intended targets? Despite the many pamphlets, leaflets, press releases and 'victory' communiqués published in several languages, who takes notice? Taiwanese authorities insist the world is listening, but the truth is that it hardly does. Taiwan's former representative in Geneva indirectly recognized this and mentioned that Taiwan needs 'branding' in Europe (interview with Peter Chang, 9 June 2004).

While Taiwan's application is based on perfectly valid legal arguments and precedents, Taiwan chooses to ignore its political dimension. In the absence of clear rules each application leads to negotiations, even more so when it is an application for 'quasi-permanent observer' status by a controversial candidate. Focusing on legal arguments at the expense of political ones can be costly: as recognized by the US State Department, Taiwan's application for membership in 2007, though expertly grounded in legal terms, negatively affected its chances of becoming an observer (*Taipei Times*, 4 April 2008).

In addition, most of Taiwan's medical arguments are unconvincing. No conclusive evidence is provided that Taiwanese people were physically affected because of exclusion from the WHO during the three emergencies Taiwan refers to in its campaign. Emotional appeals focusing on Taiwan's supposed suffering may be effective with a domestic audience but of little relevance in diplomatic terms. True, Taiwan has added more relevant and sophisticated arguments. Taiwan's former health minister noted that Taiwan took the initiative to implement 'the revised International Health Regulations one year before they came into force in 2007' but regretted that 'Taiwan continues to be excluded from the IHR notifiable disease reporting system, however, and is thus unable to immediately access information on disease outbreaks in other parts of the world or report local outbreaks to the WHO' (*Korea Times*, 4 April 2008). He cleverly concluded with a rhetorical question: 'Taiwan is doing everything in its power to engage in constructive cooperation and fulfill its responsibility so that global health security can be guaranteed. Can the same be said of the WHO?' (*Korea Times*, 4 April 2008). Chen Shui-bian also defended

> the pragmatic stance of seeking meaningful participation in the WHO. This includes participation in GOARN, WHO technical meetings and regional activities, and the International Health Regulations (IHR) mechanism. This is based on practical needs in health and disease prevention and is entirely independent of political considerations. Our appeal has already received positive feedback from a number of countries, to which we wish to express our gratitude. We hope that our friends in Europe can also continue to extend their full support.
>
> (Office of the President, Republic of China (Taiwan), 2006)

On the other hand Taiwan still clings to weak or inconsistent arguments, as detailed in the section on norms, which form the basis of the MoFA's concept papers.

Taiwan could focus on arguments that carry more weight. Should a major epidemic outbreak occur, the world would be better off if Taiwan were inside rather than outside the response system, in particular for the following reasons:

1 Viruses are mutating rapidly while global trade and travel accelerate.
2 Serious outbreaks of infectious diseases originated in China in recent years.
3 Strong and timely interventions, such as mass culling of poultry, have so far limited human casualties.
4 There is no certainty that we can avoid an epidemic of the size and severity of the 1918–19 influenza epidemic.

These arguments should easily convince global public opinion that Taiwan must be included without delay in the WHO's operational mechanisms such as the GOARN. Taiwan uses some of these arguments but usually fails to articulate them in an effective way, possibly because it is unclear what the targeted audience is. Taiwan's inclusion would not be sufficient to ensure that the world fights a massive epidemic in optimal conditions, but it would be a step in the right direction. The US, EU and Japan support Taiwan's case for inclusion.

The SARS episode and earlier failures, by signatories to international health regulations, to notify outbreaks of infectious diseases suggest that critical information is often not shared without delay. As an example, a death originally attributed to SARS in 2003 was reported in a letter to the *New England Journal of Medicine* as a case of H5N1.

> This is significant because China reported its first outbreak of H5N1 to the World Health Organisation two years later, in late 2005. The discrepancy in timelines means that the avian flu virus could have been circulating for two years in China before the alarm was raised. The country dithered similarly during the Sars outbreak; China promised such a delay would never happen again.
>
> (*Timesonline*, 3 July 2006)

Taiwan's role could be crucial in the event of a large-scale epidemic originating in China, should China not be in a position to adequately and timely report all relevant epidemiological information. Taiwan's role could then be similar to Hong Kong's role as a sentinel post. Building up on the argument, Taiwan could even suggest that Hong Kong and Macao be granted observer status on the same grounds.

But substantive collaboration is more important than formal observer status. Updated epidemiological information on outbreaks, including case definition, case management, patterns of transmission, regimens etc. are publicly available on the WHO's websites. Taiwan argues that it is not enough and wants access to technical briefings, ongoing research projects and collaborating centres (Taiwan Department of Health, undated). The other aspect of Taiwan's output is assistance to countries struck by natural or man-made disasters, discussed in Chapters 6 and 7.

Possible outcomes of Taiwan's campaign

At the time of writing Taiwan has not yet been granted observer status at the World Health Assembly but may have better chances following Ma Ying-jeou's election. In this section the domestic and external determinants of Taiwan's WHO bid and their possible consequences are reviewed. The outcome(s), it is argued here, will depend on three main factors: Taiwanese public opinion, geopolitical factors and the scale of future outbreaks of infectious diseases in East Asia.

Fatalistic attitudes among the Taiwanese would be easy to understand. Taiwan is a small country threatened by a big power. In 2005 China passed an anti-secession law to legitimize an invasion of Taiwan. Even though the US has so far discouraged China from military adventurism, there is no certainty that this will always be the case. Both the UN and the WHO campaigns have so far failed to produce results. Taiwan lost six out of 29 diplomatic allies since 2000. Taiwan is a pariah and pessimism is pervasive. In a 2006 survey, 55 per cent of respondents felt that Taiwan's status is falling and 76 per cent that 'in recent years, Taiwan's international survival space has become more and more difficult to maintain' (Taiwan Thinktank, 2006).

It is therefore remarkable that the Taiwanese massively support both the UN and the WHO campaigns. In a survey following the 2008 election, 67.8 per cent of respondents supported Taiwan to join the UN (against 6.1 per cent who opposed) and 71.3 per cent supported Taiwan's 'new government to keep promoting the policy of joining the UN' (Taiwan Thinktank, 2008). In 2004, '89.4% of respondents support Taiwan's efforts to join the WHO; only 2.7% said they did not support' and

> 86.4% of respondents expressed that, if Taiwan cannot join the WHO this year, due to the opposition from the PRC, they would support the government to continue working to join the WHO next year; only 3.6% did not support such efforts.
>
> (Taiwan Government Information Office, 14 May 2004)

In a 2007 survey, 94.9 per cent of respondents in the age group 20–29 agreed that 'Taiwan should join the World Health Organization (WHO), so as to protect the safety and health of the people in Taiwan' (Taiwan Thinktank, 2007a). But interestingly, another survey showed that while 71.2 per cent of all adults thought UN membership would be helpful to protect Taiwan's national security, only 50 per cent thought it would help promote peace across the strait (Taiwan Thinktank, 2007b).

Ignoring these feelings would be suicidal for any elected government. To some, the WHO campaign should be pursued primarily because it is a stepping stone towards independence. The campaign for observer status at the World Health Assembly does not really matter anyway. Once it is achieved, full membership of the United Nations and all its specialized agencies will ensue. To others, the WHO campaign is important in itself and will allow Taiwan to expand its international network and breathing space. More detailed surveys including rankings of motivations, attitudes regarding Taiwan's status and 'name' in WHO applications, and reasons for supporting the WHO campaign but not the UN campaign, would help understand public opinion better. What existing surveys indicate, though, is that any government has very limited room to manoeuvre.

Externally, Taiwan's dependence on US military and diplomatic support is likely to increase as China rises. The US opposes challenges to the status quo, including Taiwan's perceived moves towards independence and China's threats to take over Taiwan by force. In this environment, how is Taiwan's WHO bid perceived? For some analysts the US should support the bid to lessen cross-strait tension.

> The more Taiwan is accepted into the international community as a valuable contributor, the less legitimate is China's claim of a legal right to use force against Taiwan. Delegitimizing the use of force in the Taiwan Strait also lessens the likelihood of conflict.
>
> (Tkacik, 2004)

Whether giving Taiwan more space in the international arena will help reduce tensions in the Taiwan Strait is debatable. The WHO campaign has been promoted by pro-independence NGOs since the beginning. Many of them still see observer status at the World Health Assembly as a stepping stone towards Taiwan's independence, and so does the PRC.

Supporters of a gradual approach point to the examples of APEC and the WTO. In particular, it was argued that the flexible membership policies of the ADB, APEC and the WTO allowed Taiwan to join these organizations (Chan, 1997b). In addition, China was not a member of these organizations and therefore had to negotiate access and accept compromises (Näth, 1998).

Beijing sought to expel Taiwan from the ADB as early as 1973, though the PRC did not apply for membership until 1982. China then failed to expel Taiwan from the Bank for three reasons. ADB statutes did not specify that UN membership was a prerequisite to become a member. Requirements applicable to Taiwan's membership were different as the ROC was a founding member of the Bank. Lastly, the Republic of China's membership was geographically based on Taiwan and the other islands under its control. The PRC then tried to get Taiwan's status downgraded to associate member. The request was turned down, as the statutes of the bank do not provide for associate membership. Finally, a compromise was found and it was agreed that the Republic of China would retain membership under the name 'Taipei, China' (Chan, 1997b).

Both the PRC and the ROC became APEC members since 1991. They are represented at the same level (Ministry of Economy) but the ROC was forced to accept the name 'Chinese Taipei' (Chan, 1997b). In the case of the GATT/WTO, the Republic of China was excluded in 1972 and applied for readmission in 1990. The PRC applied for membership in 1986. Negotiations took a very long time as under the GATT and WTO rules applicants must reach agreements with each member. Many countries had reservations about China's application, but the consensus was that Taiwan could not be admitted before China. Both China and Taiwan were eventually admitted in 2001.

In all three cases Taiwan had some leverage, as China was not yet a member of these organizations. Even though the WHO offers similar flexibility in terms of membership policies, there is an important difference: Taiwan is currently out, while China is in. Taiwan was therefore unable to take advantage of WHO procedural rules to include its proposal in the agenda of the Health Assembly. A simple invitation of the Director-General to attend the Health Assembly would allow Taiwan to join as an observer, but was never extended in the absence of a consensus among members. Such a consensus might have been reached if China were not yet a WHO member.

Taiwan underlines the moral dimension of its medical and humanitarian arguments. The moral high ground Taiwan claims was very likely one of the factors that generated support from both Houses of Congress and pushed the US administration to support Taiwan's bid officially. But what is the next step? The State Department may be satisfied with gestures of little consequence, such as supporting a yearly motion, ritually voted down by the World Health Assembly. The State Department seized the opportunity of Taiwan's straying into a membership bid in 2007 to argue that its 'residual effect' would 'keep Taiwan from gaining observer status soon' and added that 'it did not pledge that the US would take concrete steps at the coming meeting to achieve that goal' (*Taipei Times*, 4 April 2008). Additional pressure from Congress is unlikely to generate State Department enthusiasm and other countries are unlikely to feel compelled to act if US diplomats do not see Taiwan's case as a priority.

US allies have provided some measure of support. Japan voted in favour of the inclusion of Taiwan's proposal in the agenda of the fifty-seventh Health Assembly. The European Parliament passed a motion supporting Taiwan's bid in 2002 but such a motion is not binding on member states and Europeans are not very familiar with the issue of Taiwan's participation in the WHO. But even if 27 votes from European countries were added to the tally, Taiwan would still fall far short of a majority at the World Health Assembly. To gain a majority, Taiwan needs significant support from developing countries. Would developing countries support Taiwan's bid in spite of China's displeasure? Would they see Taiwan as a small country bullied by a big power? Or as a rich country and a close US ally?

Taiwan has a rich man's problems. While there is no unquestionable evidence that anyone in Taiwan ever died because of exclusion from the WHO, every year in developing countries more than 15 million people die from known, curable infectious diseases. This puts Taiwan's suffering in perspective. The victimization argument may be effective with domestic audiences but is unlikely to carry much weight in the developing world. During the Taiwan debate at the fifty-seventh WHA the representative of Pakistan argued that it was 'morally wrong' to accept Taiwan in WHO

> because there are two billion people in the developing world who are deprived of any kind of health cover, hundreds of millions of people in developing countries who suffer from serious disease, tens of millions of people who die every year because of the lack of medicine. We have been in session for the past nine hours. What have we done for these people, which is the real business of this Health Assembly? I think we will be judged by this behaviour and we have spent all this time addressing the health concerns of 20 million-odd rather healthy Taiwanese.
>
> (WHO, 2004c: 33)

Another issue is that Taiwan does not seem to have many friends in the organization, in particular at WHO headquarters, who could provide tactical advice or time-critical information. It is not just that Taiwan has ignored the practical work carried out at many levels under the pretext that its representatives could not participate officially. Taiwan has also systematically tried, according to a former WHO official, to reach short-term illusory gains and in the process antagonized even potentially sympathetic insiders. Using deception to gain short-term 'victories' in terms of publicity may draw applause from a domestic audience, but is unlikely to draw effective support from within the organization and may be counterproductive over time. Similarly Taiwan cannot expect Margaret Chan, the WHO Director-General, to distance herself from the official PRC position.

Political and diplomatic processes are also driven by unforeseen events and crises, including geophysical disasters, financial crises and others. A dramatic event like a large-scale epidemic originating in China could have repercussions on the whole governance system. Hypothetically, an inadequate response by the Chinese authorities could lead to a large number of casualties worldwide and a global outcry. Taiwan might use such an opportunity to build up its case for observer status and succeed under dramatic circumstances. Taiwan failed to capitalize on SARS in 2003, but the SARS episode loomed large in the next Health Assembly and was specifically referred to by several delegates, including US Secretary for Health Tommy Thompson. The secret MoU between China and WHO, regarding the participation of Taiwanese experts in technical meetings, can be seen, at least in part, as an outcome of the SARS episode. What could be the next steps?

China's Taiwan policy has changed significantly under Hu Jintao's leadership. While Jiang Zemin pursued reunification, the administrations of former Presidents Lee Teng-hui and Chen Shui-bian moved towards independence. Hu's policy has focused on preventing Taiwan's independence (Chu and Guo, 2008).

> Eventual reunification of the country is the 'ultimate guiding principle' for the Mainland's strategy towards Taiwan, and preventing independence is the 'bottom line' of that strategy. Reunification can be postponed far into the future, but separation will never be acceptable.
>
> (Chu and Guo, 2008: 133)

Reunification was seen as realistic in the foreseeable future, so trying to induce Taiwan would not bring results. Instead, everything should be done to restrict Taiwan's international space (Chu and Guo, 2008). The Anti-secession Law is an important instrument as it mandates the PRC to respond militarily to a declaration of independence by Taiwan.

A notable change intervened with the election of Ma Ying-jeou in March 2008. Ma seeks to improve ties, ignore calls for independence and reduce cross-strait tensions. In return, he appeals to China to be sensitive to the aspirations of Taiwanese people, in particular with regard to participation in the WHO. How is China to respond?

China faces a dilemma. China can respond positively and remove at least some obstacles to Taiwan's participation in the WHO, but public opinion in China may perceive this as weakness. Or China can ignore Ma's offer and risk strengthening Taiwan's pro-independence movement, but a hard line may be detrimental to China's security (Cabestan, 2006).

If no agreement is reached earlier by the two sides, the accreditation process of Taiwanese journalists by the UN Office in Geneva ahead of the 2009 World Health Assembly could be an interesting test of China's goodwill and intentions. Will China allow the participation of all Taiwanese journalists and media? Will China allow selective participation – for instance only those who first register with authorities in Beijing?

The next question is: in what capacity would Taiwan be allowed to participate? After taking so much trouble to screen out any international NGO suspected of harbouring pro-Taiwan feelings or activities, China is unlikely to let Taiwan itself enter the WHO as an NGO. China has repeatedly said that Taiwan cannot join as a member because it is not an independent state and a UN member. Taiwan's 2007 and 2008 membership bids increased China's concern that observer status at the World Health Assembly, or 'quasi-permanent' observer status at the World Health Organization, is not Taiwan's ultimate objective, although great efforts were made in the past to defend this view publicly (Taiwan Ministry of Foreign Affairs, undated). Ironically, these efforts may have, possibly unwittingly, alarmed China even more when in a concept paper the MoFA clumsily paraphrased Burci and Vignes (2004: 22) and stated that

> It has been widely recognized that WHO's flexible procedural requirements together without any possible of a membership veto as in the United Nations' Security Council is the reason why the Organization has been the first choice for a number of countries wishing to enter the United Nations family.
>
> (Taiwan Ministry of Foreign Affairs, 2005a: 14)

In theory, China could ask the WHO to admit Taiwan as an associate member. This would be consistent with China's sovereignty claim. The move could be rationalized as the belated recognition that, because of different levels of development (objective conditions), the health priorities of China and Taiwan are different. To reinforce the argument, China could simultaneously nominate the Hong Kong SAR and Macau SAR for associate membership. The strategy would not be without risk and would provide Taiwan a stage and multiple opportunities to argue its case. Should Taiwan then annoy WHO members with its own not-so-pressing health issues or unrelated cross-strait feuds, support for Taiwan may wane. Besides, China could at any time withdraw its support for Taiwan's associate member status. In any case, Taiwan is unlikely to accept such an offer, as Premier Frank Hsieh stressed that Taiwan 'will not agree to an arrangement to become a part of the People's Republic of China in order to gain WHO membership' (*China News Agency*, 4 April 2005).

Will China agree to Taiwan's demand for 'quasi-permanent' observer status? China may want to show goodwill after years of bitter confrontation that led to increased support for independence, but China is all too aware of the potential risks. Why would Taiwan, unlike all past and present territorially-based observers, refrain from seeking membership? Taiwan tried to do just that in 2007 and 2008. Making Taiwan an observer rather than an associate member would signal that China is after all not so sure of its sovereignty claim and could reinvigorate pro-independence activists. On the other hand, as observer status is tailor-made, China could seek to minimize Taiwan's opportunities to disrupt the Health Assembly. For instance, Taiwan could be allowed to speak only on domestic health issues, and monitoring and reporting obligations under IHR. Taiwan could be denied the right to talk about anything else, reply or raise points of order. This would certainly be very frustrating for Taiwan but could help the Chinese authorities show the world that they are flexible and care for Taiwan. While a modus vivendi might be found for the coming years, a big question mark hangs over the future: what happens after 2012, when Margaret Chan's term as WHO Director-General and Ma's term as Taiwan President are over?

Before deciding on a course of action that would give Taiwan institutional grounding within the WHO, China could respond to Taiwan's insistent requests for substantive interactions, in particular participation in the GOARN and IHR reporting mechanisms. Following Taiwan's recent membership bids, China may want to test Taiwan's claim that its only motivation is the advancement of global public health before deciding on anything else.

Concluding comments and questions

The political, scientific and humanitarian norms Taiwan invokes are strong, but on further examination many of Taiwan's arguments are unconvincing. Nonetheless, invoking health as a fundamental rights issue brings Taiwan the support of legislators in the developed world and of the largest international medical associations.

China's clout and power leaves little diplomatic space for Taiwan in the international arena. Nonetheless, China strives so hard to snap any link between Taiwan and the WHO, whether through market or civil society organizations or the press and media, that China acknowledges, perhaps grudgingly, the power of non-state actors in cross-strait relations and beyond. Taiwan could under certain circumstances become an observer but its bids for WHO membership in 2007 and 2008 have heightened Beijing's anxieties and reinforced suspicions that participation in the WHO as an observer is just a step in a process and that the ultimate outcome targeted by Taiwan is full representation as a sovereign state in the United Nations.

The next two chapters again address this issue as the focus is on Taiwan's medical and humanitarian aid. What norms does Taiwan follow or refer to in its aid efforts in these fields? How does Taiwan combine these norms? What are the actors involved in Taiwan's overseas aid programmes? What are the interactions between the various actors involved? How do they link up and cooperate, not just among themselves, but also with other actors globally? In what measure does Taiwan provide aid to achieve better health outcomes for the intended beneficiaries? How far is this aid tied to the goal of observership at the WHO? How to ascertain the difference between processes and outcomes?

6 Taiwan's medical and humanitarian aid experience

Key governance elements

Introduction

The focus here is on humanitarian and medical aid provided overseas by Taiwan-based organizations. The moral, scientific and political dimensions of Taiwan's aid were introduced in Chapters 2 and 4. In addition, economic norms and arguments are also important dimensions of aid. The governance elements of norms, actors, processes, outputs and outcomes are again used here to structure and inform the discussion.

In terms of governance norms: do global norms influence Taiwan's aid providers, in particular with regard to humanitarian and medical aid? How far does Taiwan conform or comply with the evolving norms set by leading donors?

In terms of governance actors: what are the actors involved in Taiwan's medical and humanitarian aid? Are they similar to the aid actors usually found in other donor countries? Does Taiwan's unclear status bear on the various actors?

In terms of governance processes: does Taiwan's status force the government to give more leeway to non-state actors, or make the government more dependent on them? Are the various actors hampered by Taiwan's low international recognition? Do they maximize the use of instruments at their disposal?

In terms of outputs and outcomes: what are Taiwan's aid outputs and outcomes? In particular, does its unclear status lead Taiwan to deliver atypical outputs or seek outcomes that it would otherwise not be interested in?

In this chapter the stage is set with key governance elements of Taiwan's aid introduced and put in the broader perspective of global medical and humanitarian aid. The four sets of issues are then revisited and discussed in greater detail in Chapter 7.

Governance norms

The tension between political and humanitarian norms was discussed in Chapters 2 and 4 and scientific/medical/technical norms in Chapter 4. In addition to these, economic norms are introduced here.

Political norms

For a long time, global health governance hardly had anything to do with aid. The measures contained in the International Health Regulations were primarily meant to protect trade, not to improve public health in less developed countries.

With the creation of the World Health Organization the political dimensions of health were expanded as health was seen as 'fundamental to the attainment of peace and security' (WHO Constitution). Taiwan insists health is a rights issue but refers to even wider norms in the global arena, as emphasized by former President Chen Shui-bian:

> As globalization gradually links the international community together, making democracy and human rights shared values, the world's developing countries are still facing abject poverty and development challenges. Therefore, the United Nations issued the UN Millennium Declaration and the UN Development Goals as concrete solutions, and proposed a timetable to address these difficulties.
>
> (NGO Affairs Committee, 2006: 2)

Taiwan claims its aid serves Taiwan's interest and improves the well-being of populations of friendly countries. Taiwan's interest is served in several ways. Aid is supposed to improve Taiwan's image, enhance global recognition and help cement diplomatic alliances.

Transparency and accountability have gradually become important global aid norms. Following concerns over transparency in relief efforts in the aftermath of the December 2004 tsunami, these principles were re-emphasized by the OECD:

> The Principles embrace the key areas and activities where donors should work together to ensure that they support country-led anti-corruption strategies and that aid programmes do not foster corruption. Specifically, the Principles emphasize the need to support and strengthen the capacity of civil society for strengthening the demand for reform, and promoting and monitoring transparency and accountability in the fight against corruption. At the same time, they underline the need for OECD donors to work at home in their own countries on areas such as repatriation of assets, money laundering, or the ratification and implementation of the United Nations Convention against Corruption.
>
> (OECD/DAC, 2006: 3)

Taiwan claims to follow these norms. The International Cooperation and Development Fund (TaiwanICDF) defends its budget and reports its activities to the Legislative Yuan [Parliament] every year. The MoFA's budget is open to scrutiny from legislators (interview with Benjamin Liu, 22 September 2004). In addition Taiwan's Government Information Office publishes numerous accounts of Taiwan's aid programmes and activities. In contrast to other donors, Taiwan insists that its aid is not tied; recipients are not requested to source contracted goods and services from Taiwanese companies.

Scientific/medical/technical norms

There was a sea-change from minimalist nineteenth-century global health governance to the WHO's goal of 'attainment by all peoples of the highest possible level of health' (WHO Statutes, Article 1) and health has become an overarching, all-encompassing concept. Eradication and prevention became driving concepts in international health cooperation. The eradication of smallpox in the late 1970s was rightly hailed as a success that epitomized and vindicated the joint efforts of donors and health authorities in disease-endemic countries. But eradication's status as a key paradigm in international health cooperation was challenged as there were hardly any credible candidates, barring polio.

Meanwhile, medical services remained out of the reach of most people in developing countries. Therefore, emphasis was laid on making basic healthcare services available to the many people that had long been deprived of access. To this effect, common pathologies and uncomplicated cases were to be handled at the primary level and other cases referred to the secondary and tertiary levels. This had economic implications, an issue which is returned to below. Besides, essential drug model lists were established to help standardize treatments and reduce costs.

The paradigm changed again in the 1980s as infectious diseases emerged or re-emerged. While efforts to tackle the HIV/AIDS pandemic initially focused on prevention and health education, R&D-based pharmaceutical companies came up with effective treatments in a remarkably short timespan. But HIV/AIDS had by that time spread to the general population in many countries of sub-Saharan Africa, where only a very small number of patients could afford new treatments based on expensive, patented drugs.

Re-emerging infectious diseases such as malaria and TB were increasingly recognized as major threats. Resistance to chloroquine [quinine] reached such important proportions that it no longer made sense to use it as a first line treatment in antimalarial programmes in Africa. Similarly, the incidence of multidrug resistant tuberculosis (MDRTB) rose in many regions. The combination of long treatments and old drugs with heavy side-effects led many patients to discontinue treatment, thus accelerating the emergence of resistance. The situation was even bleaker for neglected diseases such as leishmaniasis or trypanosomiasis (sleeping sickness). It became clear that there would be no improvement on the infectious disease front without targeted R&D.

Humanitarian norms

Humanitarian norms were introduced and discussed in Chapter 2. The Taiwanese Red Cross is the guardian of these principles (independence, impartiality, universality and neutrality) in the context of Taiwan. Diplomatic recognition is considered by Taiwanese authorities as a prerequisite for technical cooperation, which includes medical aid, but not for humanitarian aid (interview with Stephen Lee, 21 September 2004). Beneficiaries of Taiwan's official disaster relief assistance are not required to maintain official diplomatic ties but must be 'friendly' countries. This generally means the establishment of substantive, unofficial diplomatic ties.

NGOs involved in overseas medical and humanitarian aid hold diverse views based on their underlying philosophies or religious affiliations. For instance, the Buddhist aid organization Tzu Chi emphasizes the principles of directness, priority, respect, timeliness and practicality. Directness implies a person-to-person contact between Tzu Chi volunteers and the households who need help. Priority means Tzu Chi's willingness to target people most immediately in need as resources are necessarily limited. Tzu Chi also insists on respect for the recipients:

> Wherever Tzu Chi relief workers go to help, they must respect the local customs, lifestyle, religion and cultural traditions. They should help the victims as friends and avoid being condescending. The quality of the relief supplies such as clothing, food, medicine or shelters should be of good quality, as if they were for the volunteers' own use. Finally, the relief supplies should be handed to the victims with both hands and with gratitude toward them for letting the volunteers help.
>
> (Tzu Chi, 2000)

This points to wide differences in aid norms, values and principles between the government and NGOs. As an example, the Deputy Director of the Department of Religious Affairs of the Tzu Chi Foundation explained to a South African diplomat that

> Tzu Chi's emphasis on having gratitude and respect toward the people they help, for without them, they would not be able to learn the true value of life. The director also explained that Tzu Chi does not promote religion, politics, or propaganda, and when carrying out missions, there is no giver, no receiver and no gift. The volunteers are unattached to these concepts. Instead, they will treat everyone as a brother or sister.
>
> (*Tzu Chi News*, 18 July 2004)

Local affiliates of international organizations in Taiwan refer to principles jointly defended by all member organizations. This is the case in particular of World Vision and Caritas. On its website World Vision Taiwan refers to World Vision core values:

> We are Christian
> We are committed to the poor
> We value people
> We are stewards

We are partners
We are responsive.
(World Vision, undated)

According to Father Peter Mertens, Secretary-General of Caritas-Taiwan, 'Caritas' philosophy is one of encouraging self-sufficiency. "We want human development, development of groups" … "If you give money to people, they become beggars. If you help them do what they do well, you help them become human beings"' (*Taipei Journal*, 2 February 2001). These are just the views of a few important Taiwanese NGOs and not an exhaustive coverage of the issue.

Economic norms

In the late 1940s, effectiveness became one of the key norms guiding foreign economic and financial aid in general. Aid was thought to be effective if it fostered long-term economic development, but no specific economic norms applied to medical aid. Aid was meant to accelerate economic growth, measured by macro-economic indicators. Health indicators were just outcomes of aid policies. It was not clear how the WHO's ambitious targets were to be achieved. States were expected to draw primarily on their own resources, but many newly independent countries lacked the most basic human and financial resources.

Besides political and medical dimensions, access to basic healthcare has geographical and financial aspects. People did not have access to healthcare services because no such services were available nearby or because they could not afford these services. Bilateral donors and multilateral agencies started reshaping their aid programmes alongside the access paradigm. At the same time, financial resources started dwindling as a result of structural adjustment programmes. ODA from Western countries levelled off in the 1980s, then declined in the 1990s. The shortfall could not be covered by emerging donors.

Private resources started complementing official aid and a new paradigm emerged: the age of philanthropy. Private generosity was supposed to make up for state stinginess. Private generosity involved new players and norms. Altruistic motives and humanitarian imperatives were mixed not just with national interest, but increasingly with commercial and corporate interests too. States, in particular the US, started counting as 'national' the aid provided by businesses and multinational corporations based in their own country.

Emerging and re-emerging infectious diseases forced health authorities, experts and donors to re-examine the dominant paradigm. Medical progress could no longer be a more or less natural outcome of economic development. The current norms of international medical aid and cooperation have evolved as a result of this complex history. In particular, the Commission on Macroeconomics and Health identified multidimensional links between health and poverty and established that the health status of a population is one of the main determinants of poverty. The Commission also concluded that a significantly scaled-up financial effort of donors backed by suitable policies in disease-endemic countries would yield massive economic gains (WHO, 2002d). This defined a new norm for medical aid governance. The Working Group 5 of the Commission highlighted in its report that donors should remain committed for two decades or more and obstacles to the maximization of health services should be removed, with a specific focus on health managers' skills at the district level (WHO, 2002d).

Taking stock of these evolutions the OECD stressed the necessity to invest in health in order to reduce poverty, recognizing that 'beyond its intrinsic value to individuals, health is also central to overall human development and to the reduction of poverty' (OECD/WHO/DAC, 2003: 14).

New issues arise from this paradigm shift (Thomas and Weber, 2004). As the focus intensifies on health as a *means* to achieve social and economic progress, the result may be renewed impetus to achieve measurable health outcomes. The risk is that this might also lead to lower emphasis on health as a *right*. Notwithstanding the sensitive issue of the diplomatic status of recipients, Taiwan also refers to global norms. In particular, Taiwanese authorities emphasize that 'in carrying out its international cooperation activities, TaiwanICDF remains centred on the mainstream values of the international community and aims to work in concert with international trends' and that in the pursuit of sustainable development TaiwanICDF 'will participate actively in various international sustainable development initiatives in an effort to exhibit its responsibility as a member of the global village' (TaiwanICDF, 2004: 12).

In parallel, an increasing number of diverse actors from the state, market and civil society sectors have been mobilized to this effect.

Governance actors

Global actors

As the WHO was rather restrictive in its financial support for newly independent countries, other organizations helped fill in the void, in particular UNICEF. Created in 1946 to provide relief to children in Europe, UNICEF was made a permanent UN organization in 1953. Present in 190 countries, UNICEF is a global service delivery agency with a specific mandate regarding education and children's rights. UNICEF's mission is to

> defend children's rights, help meet their basic needs, ensure their survival and increase their opportunities to flourish … respond to emergencies and strengthen the ability of children and their families to handle crises, including armed conflict, natural disaster and HIV/AIDS … advance equal rights for boys and girls and encourage their full participation in the development of their communities
>
> (UNICEF, 2003: 28)

UNICEF's contribution in the field of immunization has long been recognized. UNICEF also focuses on the prevention of HIV/AIDS among young people and help to affected children and their families. UNICEF is governed by an Executive Board of 36 members, elected by the United Nations Economic and Social Council for three-year mandates (UNICEF, 2003).

In the 1990s, the World Bank became the main donor for health projects in developing countries. At the same time, 'WHO lost ground also as a policy provider to the World Bank' (Thomas and Weber, 2004: 194). For the World Bank, 'the first priority must be to pay special attention to the needs of the poorest people in the poorest countries in the world' (World Bank, 2005: 3). In particular, the Bank is the largest global funding agency for HIV/AIDS programmes.

In 1994 the UN Economic and Social Council established a specialized organization to respond to the HIV/AIDS pandemic. The Joint United Nations Programme on HIV/AIDS (UNAIDS) claims to be 'the main advocate for global action on the epidemic' (UNAIDS, undated). Its stated purpose is to lead, strengthen and support 'an expanded response aimed at preventing transmission of HIV, providing care and support, reducing the vulnerability of individuals and communities to HIV/AIDS, and alleviating the impact of the epidemic' (UNAIDS, undated).

As the challenge of emerging and re-emerging infectious diseases seemed intractable, the Global Fund against malaria, TB and HIV/AIDS was created in 2002. This followed solemn declarations by leaders of G8 countries in 2000 in Okinawa, African leaders at a summit in Abuja, Nigeria in 2001 and a special session on AIDS at the UN General Assembly the same year. The Fund's 23-person international board

> includes representatives of donor and recipient governments, non-governmental organizations, the private sector (including businesses and foundations) and affected communities. Key international development partners of the Global Fund also include the World Health Organization (WHO), the Joint United Nations Programme on HIV/AIDS (UNAIDS) and the World Bank. The latter also serves as the Global Fund's trustee.
>
> (Global Fund, undated)

The UNHCR is responsible for the health of refugees and, in some measure, internally displaced people. Service delivery is often delegated to specialized NGOs that provide medical aid to these populations.

The role of non-state actors, including NGOs and pharmaceutical companies, was recognized early on by the WHO. The role of NGOs as health policy advisers and service delivery agencies was discussed in Chapter 4 and the role of pharmaceutical companies mentioned in Chapter 2. In contrast to generic manufacturers, R&D-based pharmaceutical companies constitute a small and exclusive club, focused on the discovery and development of new drugs. Grouped in the International Federation of Pharmaceutical Manufacturers Associations (IFPMA), these companies played key roles in norm-setting with regard to TRIPS (Trade-related aspects of Intellectual Property) and the ICH (International Conference on

Harmonisation), two international regimes which have a decisive impact on global health outcomes.

More recently, multinational companies from all sectors started paying attention to global health governance. The Global Business Coalition claims that it 'is now the pre-eminent business organization leading the business fight against HIV/AIDS and is the only business-led organization committed to harnessing the power of the business community to fight the pandemic' (Global Business Coalition, undated). Created in 1997, the GBC has over 200 members including many leading multinational corporations. The Global Business Coalition focuses on the effective provision of prevention, testing and treatment services to HIV/AIDS patients.

State actors

While multilateral agencies have gained prominence in medical aid, donor states rely primarily on bilateral cooperation. Bilateral cooperation services were created by donor countries to handle foreign aid issues. Sometimes ranked as Ministries, organizations in charge of foreign aid are more often statutory bodies, like the USAID in the US, the DfID in Britain or the GTZ in Germany. Official Development Assistance (ODA) is often channelled through one agency but there may be more than one statutory body involved. For instance, US food aid is supervised by the Department of Agriculture. EU members channel part of their humanitarian aid through the ECHO (European Community Humanitarian Office). Some donor countries set up specialized statutory bodies for medical cooperation.

The main state organizations involved in Taiwan's medical and humanitarian aid are the Taiwan International Cooperation and Development Fund (TaiwanICDF), the Ministry of Foreign Affairs (MoFA), the Department of Health (DoH) and the Council of Agriculture (CoA). Besides, a specialized unit, the Taipei Fire Department, is involved in rescue operations.

The Ministry of Foreign Affairs is involved in medical and humanitarian assistance in several ways: the MoFA oversees the operations of TaiwanICDF; the ministry's Department of International Organizations (DIO) channels the cooperation with international organizations, both governmental and non-governmental. In addition, the departments responsible for bilateral cooperation (Department of African Affairs, Department of Central and South American Affairs, Department of East Asian and Pacific Affairs) sanction loans to allies, including loans for medical infrastructure.

TaiwanICDF, a statutory body supervised by the MoFA, focuses on economic aid, which represents the bulk of its activity. In addition, TaiwanICDF inherited the mandate of providing humanitarian assistance to countries struck by disasters from one of its predecessors, the International Humanitarian Relief Fund (IHRF), created in 1988. TaiwanICDF therefore carries out aid programmes categorized as technical assistance, education and training, and international humanitarian assistance. Medical assistance projects are regarded as technical assistance missions.

TaiwanICDF's Board of Directors includes 'senior government ministers, heads of other government agencies, distinguished scholars, and leading industrialists. One-third of the Board must come from the latter two categories' (TaiwanICDF, 2004: 5). The ICDF also has a Board of Supervisors appointed, like the Directors, by the ROC Executive Yuan (TaiwanICDF, 2004).

The Department of Health's International Cooperation Bureau was set up by the Legislative Yuan. The Bureau has a small budget to fund exploratory and other missions.

> While DOH's major tasks focus on domestic health care promotion, the ICU interacts with organizations worldwide, including not only national bureaucracies, but also international governmental organizations (IGOs) and non-governmental organizations (NGOs). 'Today, the ICU also serves as a diplomatic body with a medical care focus, addressing various needs arising from epidemics, disease, calamities and public health issues worldwide'.
>
> (*China Post*, 30 April 2004)

The Agriculture and Food Agency, under the Council of Agriculture, is in charge of Taiwan's official food aid programme, started in 2002 (Chen, Wen-deh, e-mail, 18 August 2006). The Agency handles requests for food aid by foreign governments or Taiwanese NGOs, in particular for the relief of famine. The Legislative Yuan supervises the programme's budget. The Taipei Fire Brigade undertakes rescue operations in the aftermath of natural disasters. In particular, it despatched a specialized team to help find survivors after the Bam earthquake in Iran in December 2003.

Non-state actors in Taiwan's medical and humanitarian aid

Market organizations involved in Taiwan's medical cooperation and relief efforts include pharmaceutical and medical equipment companies. In addition, Taiwanese businessmen in allied and friendly countries have sometimes been enrolled in medical and humanitarian aid efforts.

Taiwanese NGOs started providing overseas humanitarian and medical assistance in the 1990s. They can be categorized in four distinct groups: Christian churches and associated hospitals; members of existing global networks; international organizations based on Taiwan religious organizations; and local NGOs actively engaged in international activities (Taiwan International Medical Alliance, 2004). Christian organizations include the Taiwan Presbyterian Church and Mackay Memorial Hospital, the Chinese Christian Medical Mission, the Hengchun Christian Hospital and Pingtung Christian Hospital, and the Taiwan Lutheran Church and ChiaYi Christian Hospital. The NGO Affairs Committee of the Ministry of Foreign Affairs lists 22 Taiwanese NGOs involved in overseas medical or humanitarian aid (NGO Affairs Committee, 2006).

Created by Master Cheng in 1966, the Tzu Chi Foundation is the largest Taiwanese charitable organization. The Foundation first targeted impoverished groups in Hualien County in Eastern Taiwan. The Foundation claims a membership of four million in Taiwan. Tzu Chi is a Buddhist organization with two main divisions, the Tzu Chi Foundation and the volunteer organization. 'The non-profit foundation alone has about 100 staff members and controls about US$0.6 billion in funds' (Huang, 2002: 3). The volunteer organization has about 10,000 commissioners worldwide. They have recruited at least 40 households each and devoted themselves to Tzu Chi's spirit and missions (Huang, 2002).

Buddha's Light International Association (BLIA) was established in Taiwan in 1991. The organization has more than 100 chapters worldwide and emphasizes social services. Other NGOs involved in overseas medical and humanitarian aid include Taiwan Roots Medical Peace Corps (TRMPC), Taiwan International Medical Alliance (TIMA), the Federation of Medical Professionals in Taiwan (FMPAT), Taipei Overseas Peace Services (TOPS) and International Action and Cooperation Team (iACT).

The FMPAT focuses on Taiwan's WHO campaign (see Chapter 4) and has not implemented medical cooperation activities, although it is planning to do so (interview with Wu Shuh-min, 23 September 2004). Taiwan Root Medical Peace Corps is a voluntary medical organization 'dedicated to improving quality of life through provision of medical services and health education' (Taiwan International Medical Alliance, 2004: 29). Created in 1995, the TRMPC decides on its missions independently but does not have an explicit operational policy. Its founder, Dr Chi-Chun Liu, insists on maximum motivation as a prerequisite. The medical professionals who join the TRMPC do not receive any form of compensation and normally pay for airfares to the countries where they intervene.

The Taiwan International Medical Alliance was founded in 2001 by medical professionals. The organization carries out several medical cooperation projects in Southeast Asia. The TIMA also intends to support the 'activities of humanitarian organisations like Oxfam and Médecins Sans Frontières' (Taiwan International Medical Alliance, 2003). The iACT was created in 2000 by a group of 'enthusiastic young professionals from various fields in Taiwan, including doctors, nurses, public health specialists, lawyers, social workers, sociologists, and anthropologists' (Taiwan International Medical Alliance, 2004: 37).

The Taipei Overseas Peace Service (TOPS) was created in 1980 as a joint effort of the China Association for Human Rights and the government of Thailand to provide services to refugees of Chinese descent in the country. Its activities now extend to refugees in Southeast Asia and Africa, regardless of their ethnic background (Taiwan International Medical Alliance, 2004). The Chinese Association for Relief and Ensuing Services (CARES) was founded in 1950 and originally focused on 'Chinese military communities' in Northern Thailand (Taiwan International Medical Alliance, 2004: 33). The CARES was also recently involved in humanitarian aid to Latin America and Turkey.

Local NGOs involved in overseas medical and humanitarian aid also include the Eden Social Welfare Foundation, the Noordhoff Craniofacial Foundation, Compassion International and the Ming Daw Culture Centre. The Noordhoff

Craniofacial Foundation and the Eden Social Welfare Foundation are more specialized and respectively focus on plastic surgery and disability. Compassion International was 'established in the summer of 1995 with ideas and projects initiated by a Buddhist master from Vietnam' (Taiwan International Medical Alliance, 2004: 26). The organization carries out projects in both Taiwan and Vietnam. Lastly, the Ming Daw Culture Centre extends medical aid to countries in Africa, Central America, the Caribbean and the Pacific.

Taiwan's humanitarian actors also include local branches of existing global networks, first and foremost the Red Cross. As Red Cross statutes only allow one national society in each country, this creates a particular difficulty for Taiwan. The Taiwanese Red Cross is officially regarded as a branch of the Chinese Red Cross but portrays itself as the Red Cross of the Republic of China, created in 1904.

World Vision Taiwan was established in 1964 as the Taiwan branch of World Vision and is linked to 109 World Vision partners. World Vision Taiwan initially focused on

> strengthening the ministries of the church in remote mountainous areas, establishing children's homes and improving medical care institutions. In its early days, World Vision Taiwan was instrumental in supporting many smaller local charities. Then, in 1990, World Vision Taiwan was upgraded from field office to full support office, a change of status which allowed the organization to be active not only at the local level in Taiwan, but also to support international projects.
>
> (Taiwan Philanthropy Information Centre, 2004)

Founded in 1968, Caritas-Taiwan is one of the organization's 162 branches. Caritas-Taiwan's international work focused on boat people in Taiwan in the 1970s and 1980s and currently focuses on refugees in Northern Thailand (Taiwan International Medical Alliance, 2004).

The Taiwan chapter of the Kiwanis was 'established in 1967, through the American Embassy' (Taiwan International Medical Alliance, 2004: 13). It is now the largest of all chapters of Kiwanis International and funds various humanitarian efforts. Founded in 1915 in Detroit, Kiwanis International is a 'global organization of volunteers dedicated to changing the world, one child and one community at a time' (Kiwanis International, 2007). The organization has nearly 600,000 members in 96 countries.

The complexity of the medical and humanitarian issues involved, the rapid evolution in norms and the increasing number of actors of various types point to another challenge: how do these actors cooperate or interact? This issue is addressed here.

Governance processes

The focus is here on governance processes in terms of linking arrangements and policy instruments as defined in Chapter 2. ODA to health has evolved rapidly and non-state actors have played increasingly important roles. Governance processes involving states in general and the Taiwanese government in particular are examined here, before focusing on non-state actors. The interactions between state and non-state actors are then highlighted.

State processes

As mentioned earlier, several IGOs are involved in global health governance, including the WHO, UNICEF and the World Bank. TDR, the Special Programme for Research and Training in Tropical Diseases, was created in 1975 to accelerate research and development efforts targeting tropical diseases. The programme, a joint effort of UNICEF, the WHO, the UNDP and the World Bank, is located at WHO headquarters and 'operates within a broad framework of intergovernmental and interagency cooperation and participation' (WHO, 1978).

The UNAIDS is another example of intergovernmental and interagency cooperation. Created in response to the HIV/AIDS pandemic, UNAIDS is co-sponsored by ten organizations: UNHCR, UNICEF, WFP, UNDP, UNFPA (United Nations Population Fund), UNODC (United Nations Office on Drugs and Crime), ILO, UNESCO, WHO and the World Bank. The creation of UNAIDS signalled a more ambitious and systematic effort by states and intergovernmental organizations to address an emerging public health crisis.

Bilateral aid remains the major component of external aid, in particular aid to the healthcare sector. Bilateral ODA to health represented 66 per cent of total ODA to health in 1996–98 (excluding bilateral contributions to UN agencies such as the WHO and UNICEF). This share increased to 77 per cent in 1999–2001 (OECD/WHO/DAC, 2003).

In 1961 Western countries and Japan set up the Development Aid Committee (DAC) within the OECD to reflect on aid policies. The Committee has 23 members. The DAC is the primary forum where aid policies are discussed, evaluated and harmonized but emerging donors are not members.

The Commission on Macroeconomics and Health prodded DAC members to look specifically at official assistance in the health sector. The DAC insisted in particular on the necessity to strengthen 'the capacity of the public sector to carry out the core functions of policy maker, regulator, purchaser and provider of health services' (OECD/WHO/DAC, 2003: 15). Aid recipients are placed at the centre of the efforts required. In addition, the DAC also recognized that coordination is crucial:

> The co-ordination of external partners, led by government, magnifies the effectiveness of development co-operation programmes not least because it encourages development agencies to reinforce and complement their programmes in support of the objectives specified in the poverty reduction strategy (PRS) and the health-sector plan.
>
> (OECD/WHO/DAC, 2003: 26)

Although medical aid to low-income countries often takes the form of grants, loans may also be considered. Loans are only counted as aid if there is a 25 per cent concessional element. To this effect, loans must be discounted at 10 per cent annually (OECD, 2001). Most of the financial aid for the healthcare sector is channelled directly to the governments of recipient countries.

The World Bank provides grants, loans, and credits to fight HIV/AIDS programmes. For the poorest countries, HIV/AIDS projects supported by the IDA can be financed wholly by grants rather than loans (World Bank, 2004). Besides, single-disease programmes run by Global Public–Private Partnerships usually mix instruments and combine cash resources with donations of patented drugs.

Taiwan implements medical and humanitarian aid projects bilaterally, in particular medical missions to diplomatic allies and soft loans for medical infrastructure development. Aid recipients must recognize Taiwan. Taiwan argues that diplomatic recognition is a prerequisite for aid because of practicalities: in the absence of full diplomatic ties, obstacles will stand in the way of effective outputs and outcomes. Taiwan rewards friends (carrots) and punishes defectors (sticks). TaiwanICDF manages medical missions, assesses the feasibility of relevant projects, funds them, staffs them and handles programme budgets. The Department of Health is represented on the board of TaiwanICDF and consulted on these projects, but has no role in the management of medical missions.

Material instruments include grants, loans and aid-in-kind. TaiwanICDF provides grants for relief in response to disasters and other humanitarian aid projects, while the MoFA handles bilateral 'soft loans'. Rescue operations are directly handled by the Taipei Fire Brigade. Material resources also include food aid. The government has sanctioned a quota of up to 100,000 tons of rice per year, distributed in particular through bilateral agreements. Taiwanese authorities also insist on the importance of human resources. Volunteers, usually recruited by the ICDF, are sent to implement medical and humanitarian assistance programmes. In addition, voluntary service overseas is an option for young Taiwanese men as an alternative to military service.

In some cases, state-to-state medical and humanitarian assistance is also implemented multilaterally. In particular, the MoFA's Department of International Organizations disburses and oversees Taiwan's official contribution to the Global Fund. The amounts spent by the MoFA on medical aid under bilateral cooperation agreements are usually not disclosed: specifically, the government does not provide a detailed breakdown by project or by country.

Non-state processes

Globally the material resources provided by NGOs for medical aid and service delivery are not insignificant, but their main contribution lies in advocacy. In particular, NGOs have kept important issues on the agenda, such as the issue of excess mortality resulting from curable diseases.

In Taiwan the Tzu Chi Foundation was a pioneer. The foundation's first overseas aid programmes were in response to a cyclone in Bangladesh and floods on the mainland. Tzu Chi then intervened in Nepal in 1992 (interview with Hsiang-Ming Hsu, 24 September 2004). Providing aid to alleviate short-term suffering led to questions over sustainability. The issue came to the fore in 1995 when the Taiwanese government requested Tzu Chi to help the families of demobilized KMT soldiers in Northern Thailand. A key issue was that the hilly areas where they were living could never provide an adequate environment for agricultural development or offer enough economic opportunities to lift them out of poverty.

Tzu Chi devised a long-term plan, focusing on the education of the younger generation, who would in turn support elder ones once they found jobs. Tzu Chi then decided to involve the Taiwanese business community in Thailand. The idea was that Taiwanese businessmen would not only help support the schools needed for the long-term success of the plan, but also eventually provide employment for the youth. Tzu Chi's policy thereafter focused on mobilizing local resources to address local needs in the countries where it intervened.

The next step was to involve overseas Taiwanese businesspeople institutionally. With members in 114 countries, Tzu Chi set up local chapters in 34 foreign countries. The first overseas branch, founded in the USA in 1985, is also the largest with 45 chapters and 50,000 members (Huang, 2002). Of these, 90 per cent are overseas Taiwanese, and the remainder usually overseas Chinese.

Interestingly, Tzu Chi's expansion 'was not a result of missionaries sent by headquarters but stemmed from spontaneous individual responses and the support of people in different countries' (Huang, 2002: 10). In case of an emergency the local Tzu Chi branch, wherever there is one, is the first one to respond. If Tzu Chi does not have a local branch or if the problem exceeds its organizational capacity, branches in neighbouring countries are called in. Among these, the branch with the most experience in emergency response takes on the coordinating role, with the support of a small team of experienced people from Taiwan (interview with Hsiang-Ming Hsu, 24 September 2004).

In countries where it had no branch or contact, Tzu Chi established partnerships with international NGOs. These included Paris-based Médecins du Monde [Doctors of the World] and CARE-France and US-based Knightsbridge International and Mercy Corps. Tzu Chi was thus able to intervene in several countries affected by major disasters, including Ethiopia in 1993, Rwanda in 1994 and Afghanistan in 1998. In such cases, Tzu Chi sent teams to assess local needs and co-funded the aid projects carried out by these various agencies. Whereas international networking and exposure to complex crises where Tzu Chi had no experience were the main reasons for these partnerships, 'consular' help was sometimes sought to smooth out visa problems (personal communication from a former executive of Médecins du Monde, 23 June 2003).

Personal contacts also helped two Taiwanese organizations involved in HIV/AIDS to set up programmes overseas as they

> were invited to China by international NGOs already established there and/or by local churches. Lourdes Home and Harmony were invited, respectively, by Misereor and Médecins Sans Frontières (MSF), and also by

> priests and nuns wishing to take action against the spread of HIV/Aids in their dioceses.
>
> (Rollet, 2005)

Church-based international networks like Caritas or World Vision generally pool resources globally and allocations are made by their respective headquarters. The primary role given to local branches seeking to get involved internationally is typically fund-raising. 'World Vision Taiwan started to join the international network of World Vision Partnership in 1990, funding emergency relief, community development and child sponsorship projects all over the world' (World Vision, undated). In particular, World Vision Taiwan's child sponsorship programme was expanded to include children overseas.

Processes involving state and non-state actors

IGOs involve non-state actors in particular through fundraising. UNICEF raises one-third of its budget from private sources, primarily through 37 National Committees. UNICEF also raises funds from a number of corporations, businesses, financial institutions and foundations (UNICEF, 2003). Similarly, the budget of the UNAIDS is financed by both state and non-state organizations (UNAIDS, undated). The Global Fund too focuses on attracting new financial contributions from state and non-state organizations. In its report of the Fund's first replenishment,

> Participants highlighted the importance of stronger engagement with the private sector and welcomed the private sector strategy note submitted to the London meeting by the Global Business Coalition on HIV/AIDS and the Private Sector Delegation to the Board of the Fund: 'Mobilizing Additional Resources for the Global Fund: A Planning Guide for the Private Sector'. The note highlights a renewed private sector commitment and the potential for increased contributions of three kinds: cash contributions, pro bono services and product contributions, and in-country co-investments and operational contributions.
>
> (Global Fund, 2005: 5)

Initiatives like the Global TB Alliance, Medicines for Malaria Venture (MMV) and DNDi (Drugs for Neglected Diseases initiative) mobilize both state and non-state actors. UNICEF has established disease-specific partnerships. UNICEF is a partner in the Global Polio Eradication Initiative along with the World Health Organization, Rotary International and the US Centers for Disease Control and Prevention (CDC).

Material resources, essentially grants and loans, are key instruments of aid to healthcare. The DAC notes that 'increased resources should come from a combination of public, private, domestic and external sources, including ODA and Global Health Initiatives (GHIs)' (OECD/WHO/DAC, 2003: 24). Grants are increasingly made through NGOs in both donor and recipient countries, as donors expect NGOs to deliver aid in a quick, effective, transparent and accountable way.

Initially NGOs accredited with the ECOSOC or the WHO observed rather than participated in substantive decision-making. A significant change happened when GPPPs were initiated following the pioneering work of Merck on onchocerciasis. In the health sector, GPPPs were usually partnerships between the WHO and one or more pharmaceutical MNC, while NGOs contributed to service delivery. Typically, GPPPs focused on the control or eradication of a single disease.

In recent years, public–private partnerships started focusing on the development of treatments and vaccines for tropical diseases for which there is no market incentive. Such partnerships rely on material instruments. Funding is key to the success of such ventures, as bringing to market a new drug or vaccine may take ten years or more. In-kind resources brought by pharmaceutical companies, in particular access to compound libraries, are no less critical to the success of these ventures. Such resources should be regarded as physical instruments, as they would be impossible to acquire at short notice.

The role of NGOs in global health governance was recognized in the decision-making structure of the UNAIDS, as 'UNAIDS is guided by a Programme Coordinating Board with representatives of 22 governments from all geographic regions, the UNAIDS Cosponsors, and five representatives of non-governmental organizations (NGOs), including associations of people living with HIV/AIDS' (UNAIDS, undated).

In engaging civil society the UNAIDS focuses on 'linkages between and among civil society, private sector, philanthropy, media, and with particular attention to organizations of people living with HIV/AIDS' (UNAIDS, undated).

The role of civil society organizations is also highlighted in the Global Fund's structure with representatives of affected communities included in its Board (Global Fund, undated). The Global Fund insists that NGOs representing targeted beneficiaries in recipient countries be involved in the programmes it supports. In addition, the Global Fund set up partnership forums 'to allow stakeholders to provide important feedback and guidance to the Global Fund on its impact in fighting these diseases' (Global Fund, undated). The Fund also established Country-Coordinating Mechanisms (CCMs) to

> develop and submit grant proposals to the Global Fund, monitor their implementation, and coordinate with other donors and domestic programs. CCMs are intended to be multi-sectoral, involving broad representation from government agencies, non-governmental organizations, community- and faith-based groups, private sector institutions, individuals living with HIV, TB or malaria, and bilateral and multilateral agencies.
>
> (Global Fund, undated)

Global Public–Private Partnerships for Health (GPPPHs) have pooled or pledged significant material resources valued at around US$2 billion (Initiative on Public–Private Partnerships for Health, 2004). Private foundations also became significant donors in the 1990s. The Bill and Melinda Gates Foundation provided support to various global health initiatives (GHI). Other foundations, including the Rockefeller Foundation, are significant donors in the field of healthcare and health policy for the developing world.

Policy dialogue is recognized as an important aid instrument, as 'it is essential to forge stronger partnerships around shared objectives and to elevate pro-poor health objectives to the top of the political agenda' (OECD/WHO/DAC, 2003: 26). High-profile shared commitments include the landmark Millennium Declaration adopted by the UN General Assembly in September 2000 and the Millennium Development Goals (United Nations General Assembly, 2000).

Several medical and humanitarian aid projects funded by the Taiwanese government were carried out in partnership with or through non-governmental organizations. Examples include Taiwan's contribution to polio eradication and Taiwan's support to AIDS prevention in Central Africa. Taiwan wanted to contribute directly to the WHO's polio eradication campaign but had to channel funds through Taiwan's Rotary Club and Rotary International. Globally, Rotary International was the main NGO involved in the effort.

The AIDS prevention project in Central Africa was part of a regional UNAIDS control project straddling Lake Chad. Interestingly, Taiwan's official contribution was channelled neither through the Chadian government nor the UNAIDS, but through an NGO: CARE-France. The project was approved and overseen by the Legislative Yuan. The collaboration resulted from personal contacts between the Director of CARE-France and Taiwanese authorities through the Tzu Chi Foundation (interviews with Hsiang-Ming Hsu, 24 September 2004 and Philippe Lévêque, Paris, 10 June 2005). The MoFA contributed US$1.02 million to CARE-France for an AIDS prevention programme in Chad over three years (2001–04).

In the 1990s the MoFA focused primarily on humanitarian and relief organizations. The Ministry facilitated their work and enrolled them in its disaster response diplomacy. Taiwanese humanitarian NGOs responded to a range of emergencies, from earthquake or hurricane relief in Central America to AIDS in Chad or Liberia, or refugees in Macedonia. It is not clear whether the MoFA supported humanitarian NGOs financially, as there was little transparency in the disbursement of government aid funds. But government officials acted as facilitators and focused on harvesting the 'goodwill' dividends generated.

Before his election, Chen Shui-bian made the case for a diplomacy based on human rights, as explained in Chapter 3. NGOs across all sectors would help expand Taiwan's diplomatic space. As part of its strategy to push Taiwanese NGOs to affiliate with UN-accredited INGOs, the MoFA identified medical and humanitarian assistance as one of four fields where it would offer NGOs sponsorship for overseas training. The Ministry also coordinated NGO participation in specific humanitarian assistance projects.

Emergency response projects may be initiated by state or non-state organizations, or jointly. In particular, TaiwanICDF 'works with NGOs in the evaluation, implementation and supervision of various projects. In addition, the ICDF is helping to design projects and is looking for further cooperative opportunities with NGOs' (TaiwanICDF, 2004: 17). Food aid is sometimes distributed through Taiwanese NGOs.

The Taiwanese government has often used the Red Cross channel to deliver aid overseas. Although the Taiwanese Red Cross was long confined to domestic issues, the situation changed in 1991, when the government channelled relief grants to former Soviet republics through the society (interview with Christian Li, 22 September 2004).

At a seminar on foreign aid organized by the Ministry of Foreign Affairs Tim Shao, president of World Vision Taiwan, called for NGO-government partnerships and argued that

> the Ministry of Foreign Affairs' NGO International Affairs Committee … should seek active cooperation with the Taiwan Overseas Aid and International Development Alliance (TOAID) in the following respects, Shao said. 'First, we can work together on overseas projects, meaning the government could set up its policy and the NGOs could help to implement related projects.'
>
> (*Taipei Times*, 21 December 2000)

NGOs are not necessarily limited to the role of implementing agencies. At the same seminar, Sister Emma Lee of Caritas-Taiwan ROC insisted that

> sometimes NGOs could carry more weight than the government, adding: 'There are indeed times when NGOs can help solve problems in ways the government can't.' … For instance, after Taiwan withdrew from the UN in the early 1970s, UN officials had difficulty visiting Taiwan in their official capacity to deal with the inflow of Vietnamese refugees to Taiwan's offshore islands that was triggered by the Vietnam War. 'So UN officials came to Taiwan in a private capacity and worked in our office to complete thousands of refugee settlement cases,' Lee said.
>
> (*Taipei Times*, 21 December 2000)

Caritas-Taiwan's programmes for Vietnamese refugees from 1975 and 1986 involved not only the UNHCR, but also the US and Canadian Bureaus of Immigration (Taiwan International Medical Alliance, 2004).

The physical instruments the Taiwanese government uses include the organization of transport for goods and teams. To facilitate access, Taiwanese diplomats also help organize visas. As an example, Tzu Chi reported that Taiwan's diplomatic links with Macedonia had a direct impact on its operations:

> On April 13, Tzu Chi headquarters dispatched a team to Macedonia to join a special group from the Taiwanese Ministry of Foreign Affairs. Their goal was to identify the needs of the refugees and devise a proper plan to help them.… Because Macedonia has diplomatic relationships with Taiwan, its Ministry of Foreign Affairs invited Tzu Chi, World Vision Taiwan, the

> Taiwan Red Cross, and several other local charity groups to set up field hospitals in western Macedonia and to provide relief supplies.
>
> (Tzu Chi, 1999)

With regard to material instruments, Taiwan Roots Medical Peace Corps negotiates directly with partner organizations in aid recipient countries, but solicits funds from the public and the government for its operating and logistical expenses and in-kind donations from pharmaceutical and medical equipment companies. Tzu Chi funds its relief operations through appeals to members and does not solicit funds from the government but sometimes distributes food aid given by the Council of Agriculture.

In terms of symbolic instruments, the MoFA publicizes not only humanitarian and medical aid programmes run by state organizations, but also NGO programmes. Wherever possible, MoFA highlights its role as a facilitator. As an example,

> Jewel Howard Taylor, First Lady of Liberia, came to visit the Tzu Chi Taipei branch office on November 8. On behalf of her people, she expressed sincere gratitude to Tzu Chi for sending a forty-foot container of clothes to Liberia.... President Taylor of Liberia came to Taiwan on November 5 for a week-long visit. Before their arrival, Mrs. Taylor expressed her wish to visit Tzu Chi, but due to their extremely tight schedule, she could not visit Master Cheng Yen in Hualien. Thus, the Ministry of Foreign Affairs arranged for her visit to the Tzu Chi Taipei branch office.
>
> (Tzu Chi, 1997)

Humanitarian organizations and programmes featured prominently in a recent government publication (NGO Affairs Committee, 2006). The Taiwanese government insists that it is always ready to assist humanitarian NGOs in responding to overseas emergencies (interview with Michel Ching-long Lu, 21 September 2004).

Instruments can be combined. In particular, a new modus operandi emerged in recent years. Taiwanese NGOs and the government responded quickly to assist victims of the September 11 attacks in New York and of hostilities in Afghanistan in 2001 and Iraq in 2003. Aid operations to both countries were organized by the MoFA as joint programmes with NGOs under the label: 'Love from Taiwan'. The Taiwanese government organized the transport of relief goods and volunteer teams provided by NGOs. But actual transportation was done by Taiwanese airlines, primarily China Airlines and Eva Air. China Airlines transported relief goods to Jordan in 2003 for delivery to Iraq. In particular, the MoFA organized a meeting in March 2003 to coordinate assistance from all sectors to Iraq:

> Foreign Affairs Minister Eugene Chien, Executive Yuan Secretary-General Liu Shih-fang and officials from the Ministry of the Interior, the Department of Health and the Council of Agriculture, as well as lawmakers Parris

> Chang of the ruling Democratic Progressive Party and Sun Ta-chian of the opposition People First Party all attended the meeting. Representatives from World Vision Taiwan, the Buddhist Tzu Chi Compassionate Relief Foundation, the Taiwan Roots Medical Peace Corps, the Republic of China Red Cross and the Eden Welfare Foundation, China Airlines, EVA Airways and Yangming Marine Transport Corp., among others, were also present to hear briefings by relevant government officials on their aid operations.
>
> (*Health Taiwan*, 28 March 2003)

In 2006 yet another umbrella organization was created: Taiwan International Health Action (TaiwanIHA). It is unclear how governmental or non-governmental organizations are involved. TaiwanIHA's organizational chart only refers to 'two conveners, two deputy conveners and an executive director' and a 'national policy adviser to the president' (TaiwanIHA, 2007a). The website does not mention the institutional affiliations of the conveners and co-conveners but states that 'the organization receives support and cooperation from the Department of Health and Ministry of Foreign Affairs' (TaiwanIHA, 2007a). TaiwanIHA takes credit for aid operations after the 2004 tsunami and the Kashmir earthquake in 2005. TaiwanIHA also appears to 'promote Taiwan and its position in the field of medicine internationally' in other ways and in particular sponsored the twenty-eighth World Congress of Internal Medicine, hosted in Taipei in 2006, noting that 'the International Society of Internal Medicine (ISIM), a very important international medical organization established in Switzerland in 1948, has 59 state members and 3000 individual members' (Taiwan Ministry of Foreign Affairs, 2006).

Governance outputs and outcomes

Outputs and outcomes in global assistance to health

While official aid rose in the early 2000s in line with commitments to achieve the Millennium Development Goals, ODA fell to US$103.7 billion in 2007, down from a high of US$107.1 billion in 2005 (OECD, 2008a). The World Bank (IDA), the leading donor of ODA to health for the period 1996–98, was subsequently overtaken by the US (OECD/WHO/DAC, 2003).

WHO's output, as detailed in Chapter 4, consists primarily of research and technical guidelines. UNICEF's output is not limited to healthcare but focuses in particular on immunization. Immunization is also an entry point leading to the delivery of other services: 'At vaccination sessions we may distribute insecticide-treated mosquito nets to help protect families from malaria, or provide Vitamin A supplements, which help children survive when they fall sick' (UNICEF, undated). UNICEF's contribution to polio eradication can be measured by its outputs:

> UNICEF has delivered over 10 billion doses of oral polio vaccine (OPV) to over two billion children over the last fifteen years. We help countries to maintain a 'cold-chain' of refrigeration units and ice-boxes to protect the

> vaccine until it reaches children living in remote regions. Along with our partners, we also work with traditional and religious leaders to help organise immunization campaigns and mobilize communities to participate. A fundamental part of our work includes a drive to increase access to routine immunization against polio and other childhood diseases.
>
> (UNICEF, undated)

Immunization represented 21 per cent of UNICEF direct programme assistance in 2003 and HIV/AIDS 9 per cent (UNICEF, 2003). In terms of physical outputs, UNICEF reports that

> More than 100 million infants are immunized each year. Immunization rates for the six major vaccine-preventable diseases rose from under 10 per cent in the 1970s to 76 per cent in 2002. East Asia and the Pacific regions improved immunization coverage from 38 per cent in 1980 to almost 90 per cent since 1990. Coverage in Latin America and the Caribbean increased from 38 per cent in 1980 to about 87 per cent in 1999.
>
> (UNICEF, 2006a)

The UNAIDS focuses on 'leadership and advocacy for effective action on the epidemic, strategic information to guide efforts against AIDS worldwide, tracking, monitoring and evaluation of the epidemic and of responses to it' (UNAIDS, undated). The World Bank supports programmes targeting infectious diseases, health systems performance, child health, nutrition and reproductive health (World Bank, 2004). The World Bank is the largest multilateral donor to healthcare in developing countries.

One of the most notable outcomes in terms of global health governance was the eradication of smallpox, officially declared by the thirty-third World Health Assembly in 1980. Polio is the only other disease for which eradication appears to be in sight. Only four countries reported indigenous polio transmission in 2005, down from six in 2004. But polio outbreaks recently occurred in particular in Nigeria, Indonesia, Yemen and the Horn of Africa (WHO, 2006b).

UNICEF claims that the massive immunization drive spearheaded by the agency 'has saved over 20 million lives in the last two decades. Distribution of high-dose vitamin A capsules has averted an estimated 1 million child deaths between 1998 and 2000' (UNICEF, 2006a). UNICEF is committed to 'protect all children from polio by immunizing every child until the disease is eradicated' (UNICEF, undated). A global leader in vaccine supply, UNICEF claims to reach 40 per cent of the world's children but also notes that 'every year, more than 2 million children die from diseases that could have been prevented by inexpensive vaccines' (UNICEF, undated). The World Bank also pays attention to outcomes. Since 1998 the Bank has put more emphasis on

> evaluating the results of its lending programs in terms of how they impact on people and their needs, rather than by measuring input levels. The Bank

> has developed several tools to carry out this task. These include evaluations that focus on the effectiveness of individual projects and more wide-ranging reviews which look at the Bank's work in whole countries and whole economic or social sectors of operation.
>
> (World Bank, undated)

To this effect the World Bank writes implementation completion reports, project performance assessment reports, impact evaluation reports and inspection panel reports for individual projects. For a broader view, the World Bank also carries out country assistance evaluations, sector and thematic reviews, and process reviews (World Bank, undated).

The Global Fund too focuses on the effectiveness of its delivery mechanism. The Fund emphasizes the need to scale up funding and focus on interventions which have been proven effective. In addition, the Global Fund does not disburse funds until there is evidence that progress is made and highlights that 'initial disbursements are particularly small. Grant recipients must strengthen program capacity and prepare procurement plans to trigger future disbursements for the purchase of medicines' (Global Fund, 2006b).

The contribution of Global Public–Private Partnerships for Health (GPPPHs) can be measured by 'the roughly US$2 billion so far collectively pledged to new non-profit ventures in the last five years'. But while it is claimed that 'In just a few years the most mature of these ventures have built up sizeable portfolios of potential products for their target diseases', it is also recognized that 'it is too early to immediately expect licensed successes from these new efforts' (Initiative on Public–Private Partnerships for Health, 2004).

Between 1975 and 2004, only 1 per cent of new drugs marketed targeted tropical infectious diseases and tuberculosis (Chirac and Torreele, 2006). In response to criticism from civil society organizations, several pharmaceutical companies have re-committed to R&D targeting infectious diseases. In addition, initiatives including the Global TB Alliance, the Medicines for Malaria Venture (MMV) and the Drugs for Neglected Diseases initiative (DNDi) have targeted infectious diseases and developed R&D pipelines.

Taiwan's medical and humanitarian aid to developing countries: outputs and outcomes

Not all of Taiwan's humanitarian and medical aid activities and programmes target developing countries. For instance the Tzu Chi Foundation runs several free clinics in the United States, which serve disadvantaged populations, notably in New York and Los Angeles. The focus here is on aid provided by Taiwanese organizations to developing countries.

In December 2003, the Taipei Fire Brigade sent a rescue team to help find survivors of the Bam earthquake in Iran. Taiwan's contribution also includes aid-in-kind such as the technical aid provided by the volunteers it sends overseas or the food provided by its aid programme. TaiwanICDF's input 'focuses on providing emergency assistance to friendly and allied nations following natural disasters. The help consists of grassroots medical, health and nutritional assistance' (TaiwanICDF, 2004: 16). TaiwanICDF grants for humanitarian aid projects amounted to more than US$1.2 million in 2003 (TaiwanICDF, 2004) but only US$400,000 in 2007 (TaiwanICDF, 2008).

The projects funded in 2003 included medical assistance for the Tibetan community in India, a TB project in the Altai region of Russia, a mobile hospital project in Mongolia, emergency regional support in response to SARS, medical assistance to Gambia, the Philippines, Sri Lanka and Chinese refugees in Northern Thailand, and the 'Love from Taiwan' operation in Iraq. Medical services account for 72 per cent of the humanitarian assistance provided by TaiwanICDF and emergency relief for 20 per cent. Geographically, 74 per cent of international humanitarian assistance provided by TaiwanICDF went to Asia, 16 per cent to Europe, 8 per cent to Africa and 2 per cent to Latin America (TaiwanICDF, 2004).

Taiwan spent 0.13 per cent of GNI on official development assistance in 2007 (OECD, 2008a). Unfortunately, specific figures for medical aid and disaster relief are not reported on a regular basis. Besides, the figures reported by various authorities are contradictory (see Table 6.1)

In the absence of details and explanations, these aggregate figures do not make much sense and lack credibility. The figures provided by TaiwanIHA included private contributions. The study commissioned by the Department of Health was the only one to provide some information on the methods and a yearly breakdown. It was compiled on the basis of information publicly available from various government and private organizations and a 'survey of 21 large hospitals and 20 private organizations' and the figures 'included training of medical workers and donation of medical supplies and equipment' (*Free China Journal*, 6 August 2004). The study reported yearly figures as follows (see Table 6.2).

With regard to humanitarian operations, Taiwan was involved in particular in responses to Hurricane Mitch in Central America in 1999, the Salvador earthquake in 2001 and the Indian Ocean tsunami in 2004. But Taiwan regrets that it could not help in the case of an earthquake in Turkey in 1999, as its

Table 6.1 Official medical and humanitarian assistance: select figures

Source	*Period*	*Nature*	*Amount (US$m)*
Taiwan Department of Health (2003)	1996–2002	Medical assistance	139
Taiwan CDC (2005)	1995–2004	Medical assistance	233
Taiwan MoFA (2005b)	1995–2003	Medical and humanitarian assistance	120
Taiwan IHA (2007a)	1997–2006	Medical and health emergency aid (not including volunteer medical care)	450

Table 6.2 Taiwan's official international medical assistance and cooperation (in US$)

1996	*1997*	*1998*	*1999*	*2000*	*2001*	*2002*
7,035,119	7,965,963	26,824,444	19,234,806	27,544,768	28,168,960	22,040,700

Source: Taiwan Department of Health (2003).

'experienced medical teams were not allowed to assist the rescue efforts; this would not have been the case if Taiwan was able to work through the WHO to dispatch medical aid' (Taiwan Ministry of Foreign Affairs, 2005b: 10). In Macedonia in 1999 Taiwan responded to a refugee crisis. Taiwan quickly announced an impressive aid package of US$300 million for Kosovo and sent a team of officials and volunteers to Macedonia to help look after refugees from Kosovo. Reports also mentioned Taiwan's official support for Afghan refugees, and a government donation of US$17 million, but it is not clear over what period (Fanchiang, 11 April 2003).

Of the 133 Taiwan overseas volunteers sent by TaiwanICDF since 1997, 13 per cent worked in medical services (TaiwanICDF, 2008). TaiwanICDF used to run medical missions in four African countries (Burkina-Faso, Chad, Malawi and São Tomé and Príncipe) but the medical missions in Chad and Malawi were terminated following the severance of diplomatic ties.

In Burkina-Faso, the medical mission provides medical services at L'Hôpital de la Liberté [Friendship Hospital] at Koudougou 'offering knowledge and technology transfers to boost the medical standards of the hospital' (Taiwan ICDF, 2004: 38). In Chad, TaiwanICDF provided services to L'Hôpital de la Liberté [Freedom Hospital] in N'Djamena and offered 'guidance in the hospital's surgical and gynaecological departments, raising medical standards' (Taiwan-ICDF, 2004: 38). In Malawi, TaiwanICDF built a hospital in Mzuzu described as 'the brainchild of the Taiwan government' (Fanchiang, 11 April 2003), reportedly at a cost of US$18 million (*Central News Agency*, 7 July 2002). In São Tomé and Príncipe, TaiwanICDF assists through 'a variety of medical technology services and ... the adoption of new management practices' (TaiwanICDF, 2004: 41) and previously helped set up a malaria control project. TaiwanICDF does not disclose the amounts spent on medical missions but yearly expenses were estimated to average US$500,000 per mission (telephone interview with Yan-di Chang, 25 October 2004).

The MoFA contributed US$1 million to the Global Fund in 2002 and another US$1 million in 2004. The MoFA also contributed US$1.02 million to CARE-France over three years (2001–04) for its AIDS control programme in Chad, designed to "help enhance Chad people's alertness against AIDS and improve their hygienic conditions", according to a joint statement by Taiwan's Vice Foreign Minister Wu Tzu-dan and Care France chairman Marina de Brantes' (*Agence France-Presse*, 12 November 2001).

The Council of Agriculture does not release all of the 100,000 tons of rice earmarked for food aid but usually donates 20,000 to 30,000 tons annually

(W. D. Chen, e-mail, 18 August 2006). The council reported donating 56,312 tons of rice under the programme in 2004 (Council of Agriculture, 2004). Food aid is sometimes channelled bilaterally, as in the case of former diplomatic allies Malawi and Liberia (Department of Humanitarian Affairs, 1997).

Food aid is also channelled through NGOs. As an example, Taiwan Rotarians delivered food aid to Southern African countries struck by famine. One of the largest food aid operations was run by Tzu Chi in Indonesia:

> Tzu Chi Foundation in Taiwan solicited 50,000 metric tons of rice donated by the Council of Agriculture, Executive Yuan of Taiwan. The rice aid distribution is a large-scale relief project aimed at providing food assistance to impoverished communities by distributing free rice to these areas. The project covers vast areas that require considerable amount of human resources and collaboration. To support this cause, many Chinese enterprises based in Jakarta have been whole-heartedly involved in finding areas to conduct the distribution and bringing the rice to these areas.
>
> (*Tzu Chi News*, 1 June 2003)

Such programmes are not always successful, as in the case of food aid to Iraq:

> The ministry, in a bid to help the Iraqi people suffering from war, worked with the Hashemite Jordan Charity Organization (HAJCO) to transport 5,000 tonnes of rice to Iraq in 2003. While 1,000 tonnes of the food aid were sent to Iraq, 4,000 tonnes of the consignment were stored at Jordan's Aqaba Port for more than a year. 'The 4,000 tonnes of rice, which is worth US$4 million, turned stale after being stored at the port for more than a year. HAJCO, without informing the MOFA, sold the rice as fodder for US$600,000 on auction,' ministry spokesman Michel Lu said yesterday. The ministry has expressed its discontent with the Jordanian government and HAJCO over the charity's 'improper act' of selling Taiwan's food donation, Lu said.
>
> (*Taipei Times*, 24 February 2005)

Taiwanese businesses also contribute to aid programmes in kind. As an example, it was reported that 'the foreign ministry plans to donate five million Taiwan-manufactured condoms to Liberia' (*Taipei Times*, 1 November 2000). The Government Information Office also stated that aid supplies were provided to Afghan refugees with the support of the Taiwan Pharmaceutical Manufacturers' Association and the Taiwan Medical Equipment Manufacturers' Association (*Taiwan Headlines*, 11 December 2001).

NGOs, sometimes supported by the government, run a wide range of programmes. The TRMPC initially focused on providing medical services to indigenous communities lacking access to existing healthcare facilities in the mountain areas of central Taiwan. At the request of the government, the TRMPC conducted its first overseas mission in 1999 to assist refugees from Kosovo. The Taiwanese group established a base in the Stankovec refugee camp in Northern Macedonia. TaiwanIHA reported that 'as the only medical team from Asia, TRMPC provided comprehensive care for approximately 40,000 refugees' (TaiwanIHA, 2007b: 26). Press reports added that their contribution was widely noticed by the international community. The TRMPC has since assisted populations in several Asian, African and Latin American countries. The projects run by iACT include medical and legal services for migrant workers in Taiwan and the training of Tibetan doctors in Nepal. In addition, iACT studied the feasibility of CARE-France's AIDS prevention programme in Chad, supported by the MoFA (Taiwan International Medical Alliance, 2004). The Taiwanese Red Cross responded to overseas emergencies in Rwanda (1994), Macedonia (1999), Afghanistan (2001) and to the Bam earthquake in Iran in 2003 (interview with Christian Li, 22 September 2004).

Tzu Chi intervened in nearly 30 countries since 1991. Large numbers of volunteers are involved but the organization does not provide financial data for its aid programmes. The amounts are certainly significant. Tzu Chi reportedly gives US$40 million every year in charity (Huang, 2002). In one instance, Tzu Chi was reported to have given US$773,000 to Ethiopia through Médecins du Monde (Huang, 2002).

Material resources raised by humanitarian organizations in response to overseas disasters have increased in recent years. In particular,

> In December 2004, following the devastating tsunami produced by a major earthquake off the coast of Indonesia, relief agencies in Taiwan initiated fundraising, with the Buddhist Compassion Relief Tzu Chi Foundation raising NT$2.4 billion in Taiwan alone, while the Red Cross Society of R.O.C. raised NT$730 million and World Vision Taiwan raised NT$630 million. That three relief agencies raised public donations totalling over US$100 million in a country of some 20 million citizens amazed the international community and raised interest about the development of Taiwan's civil society.
>
> (NGO Affairs Committee, 2006: 14)

Financial data for medical assistance by Taiwanese NGOs were recorded for the years 1996–2002 in the Department of Health study (see Table 6.3).

The Taiwanese government was involved through CARES, a quasi-governmental NGO, in projects to support demobilized KMT soldiers and their families in Northern Thailand. In 1995 Tzu Chi was brought in because of prob-

Table 6.3 International medical assistance by Taiwanese non-state actors (in US$)

1996	*1997*	*1998*	*1999*	*2000*	*2001*	*2002*
3,162,974	3,680,867	5,841,951	5,183,458	4,732,163	7,476,078	6,135,905

Source: Taiwan Department of Health (2003).

lems with the projects implemented there. Other Taiwanese NGOs also focused on the region, including the TRMPC, Caritas-Taiwan and Pingtung Christian Hospital.

In response to the December 2004 tsunami, Vice Premier Yeh Chu-lan said that Taiwan's government 'decided to boost its aid offer from US$5 million to US$50 million, including US$20 million worth of rice, US$15 million worth of medical supplies and US$15 million in community and harbor reconstruction' (*Asia Pulse*, 3 January 2005). Taiwanese NGOs, notably Tzu Chi, also provided relief, in particular to Aceh province. The government reported that altogether 'Taiwan sent 511 volunteers and medical workers to disaster areas in Indonesia, Thailand, India and Sri Lanka', but acknowledged that 'most were affiliated with NGOs' (NGO Affairs Committee, 2006: 66).

The lack of data makes it difficult to assess the impact of Taiwan's medical and humanitarian aid. It was argued that, notwithstanding obstacles, Taiwan contributed to the Millennium Development Goals:

> In view of Taiwan's diplomatically isolated position in the world, its NGOs play an important role in its overseas aid programs and efforts to advance the objectives of the MDG program. Nevertheless, despite the notable contributions made by Taiwanese NGOs, in many instances they can provide assistance only on a short-term basis. It is only when Taiwan is fully acknowledged on the international stage that it will be able to systematically make the larger contribution to the Millennium Development Goals that its economic strength warrants.
>
> (*Free China Journal*, 6 August 2004)

Outcomes Taiwan expects include the recognition of its contributions. Taiwan's government often claims that its aid operations are widely noticed and appreciated:

> Through humanitarian work, NGOs in Taiwan have received recognition domestically and internationally, helping Taiwan to gain opportunities to participate in events and activities around the world. As globalization increases interdependence between each country, Taiwan's future is intertwined with the rest of the world. The participation of Taiwan NGOs in international affairs makes them an important partner that cannot be overlooked in diplomatic efforts.
>
> (NGO Affairs Committee, 2006: 112–14)

In addition, the emphasis is on Taiwanese NGOs making their way to the UN. In December 2003, the DPI recognized Tzu Chi as an NGO with a significant information programme on issues of interest to the United Nations. The step was welcome by Tzu Chi: 'The new NGO status will help Tzu Chi volunteers on international relief missions in the future' (*Tzu Chi News*, 15 December 2003).

Humanitarian diplomacy can target multiple outcomes. In particular, the MoFA expected that Taiwan's contribution to the AIDS project run by CARE-France in

Chad 'would be a plus either in cementing ties with Chad, Taipei's bid to join non-governmental organisations and in Taipei's goal of making a greater contribution to the international society' (*Agence France-Presse*, 12 November 2001).

World Vision Taiwan also emphasizes the perception of its programmes by public opinion in Taiwan and their potential impact on the island's diplomatic situation:

> World Vision Taiwan endeavors to be one of the first national offices that respond to international emergencies by appealing to the public and delivering donations. Relief, rehabilitation and practical prevention against disasters all receive proper attention in the global service of World Vision. The Taiwan public becomes the witness of such efforts, and the international attention to the island's compassion in turn benefits the country itself in terms of diplomacy.
>
> (World Vision, undated)

Concluding comments and questions

Aid norms in the healthcare sector have evolved rapidly. Non-state actors, primarily pharmaceutical companies and medical NGOs, have gained prominence and influence. The sector has been rich in new partnerships and creative arrangements between state, market and civil society organizations. Global actors are paying more attention to outcomes than they did in the past.

Taiwan's contribution in terms of medical and humanitarian aid raises several issues. How far does it conform to changing norms in medical and humanitarian aid? Is the nature of aid actors different in the case of Taiwan as the island lacks international recognition? Are aid processes affected by Taiwan's unclear status? These issues are examined in the next chapter.

7 Taiwan's medical and humanitarian aid experience

Discussion

Introduction

The findings highlighted in Chapter 6 are discussed here. Key governance elements of Taiwan's medical and humanitarian aid were introduced in the previous chapter and put in the broader perspective of the global aid system. In this chapter the various elements of governance systems identified in Chapter 2 again serve as a guide to the analysis. The significance of Taiwan's initiatives and experiences in the field of medical and humanitarian aid to developing countries is assessed, as is their relevance to the outcomes Taiwan targets.

Governance norms revisited

Political norms

During the Cold War, Western countries distributed foreign aid to lure developing countries away from communism. After the Cold War, alignment with the US-led Western Alliance was replaced with democratic credentials and the promotion of human rights as standards of 'expected recipient behaviour'. Countries with good records in these areas were praised and led to believe that they would be preferential beneficiaries of the largesse of OECD donors. These words of encouragement may have been more symbolic instruments than a reflection of actual aid disbursements: even countries which strongly emphasized the importance of democracy and human rights kept giving significant amounts of aid to undemocratic regimes or regimes with poor human rights records (Omoruyi, 2001).

The political norms Taiwan follows in this regard do not contradict what OECD/DAC donors recognize as acceptable. The only difference lies in the specific objectives pursued by Taiwan. Each donor state has its specific objectives. Whether or not recognized as such by other states and the international community in general, Taiwan in this regard behaves like a state.

Taiwanese authorities also claim to abide by the principles of transparency and accountability. While significant changes have occurred since 2000, some sensitive information is still not disclosed to the public. The term transparency is used here 'to describe those policies that are easily understood, where information about the policy is available, where accountability is clear, and where the citizens know what role they play in the implementation of the policy' (Finkelstein, 2000: 1). The issue is discussed below in the section on political/economic norms.

Humanitarian norms

NGOs hold diverse views on aid norms. Some focus on improving access to healthcare and providing basic relief or longer-term development aid to populations in distress or affected by crises, while others argue that Taiwan's difficult position in the international arena should be taken into account. All the persons interviewed for this research stated that they would welcome Taiwan's admission to the WHO, but not all agreed that medical or humanitarian aid projects should be designed and implemented to maximize impact on the WHO campaign.

Political and humanitarian norms combined

State interests do not necessarily coincide with universal principles. States use aid to advance their own interests and according to realists this is all that really matters. In contrast, liberals argue that the purpose of foreign aid is to enhance the overall progress of mankind, for instance through economic development or the promotion of human rights. In the pursuit of state interests, each donor has its own philosophy and priorities. Donors to African countries were found to have diverse motivations (Omoruyi, 2001). Whereas France seemed to be driven by '*besoin de rayonnement*', Denmark was found to be primarily motivated by humanitarian concerns, Japan by its drive for permanent UN Security Council membership, and the US by a mix of humanitarian concerns and commercial and security interests (Omoruyi, 2001).

Like the US, Taiwan strongly prioritizes aid to close diplomatic allies. At the same time, the US gave substantial amounts of aid to alleviate the famine in North Korea and provided aid to Iran in the aftermath of the Bam earthquake in December 2003. Due to its precarious geopolitical situation, Taiwan cannot afford to provide aid to hostile countries. To ensure Taiwan's ODA rewards only allies, loans given as aid are immediately due if the recipient country breaks diplomatic links with Taiwan but this does not apply to grants earmarked for humanitarian aid (interview with Stephen Lee, 21 September 2004).

Taiwan's motivations are as diverse and ambiguous as those of other donors. On the one hand, Taiwan refers to universal principles and highlights the needs of less privileged people. On the other hand, Taiwan spells out clearly its objective of global recognition. The only difference is that, in the case of Taiwan, the need is not for increased grandeur, *besoin de rayonnement*, or the status associated with permanent membership of the UN Security Council. Taiwan's efforts in this regard are simply predicated on the right to exist in the international arena, i.e. survival as a state.

The forms that this demand implies were explored in Chapter 4. To raise its global status, Taiwan consistently refers to its aid effort as an important component of the equation. The Taiwanese government emphasizes in particular that its medical and humanitarian aid to developing countries should be acknowledged.

Political and medical norms combined

Taiwanese authorities take seriously their claim that health is a universal right and have introduced a comprehensive health insurance scheme, which they argue is the most progressive in Asia. The scheme guarantees access to healthcare for all people in Taiwan. Health as a fundamental right also appears to be a slogan that serves Taiwan's interests well. When Taiwanese officials insist that health is a universal right, they do not clearly translate their vision into medical programmes for the developing world. Aid officials appear to refer only rhetorically to the momentum created by the Millennium Declaration, the Commission on Macroeconomics and Health and debates about aid policies among OECD/DAC members.

Economic norms

Taiwan emphasizes that from the 1940s to the 1960s it was a recipient of economic aid provided by the US. The implicit norm Taiwan refers to is reciprocity. Taiwan benefited from ODA and now wants to give back. But Taiwan's aid story is not as simple as the narrative they suggest. In the months after Japan surrendered, the US increasingly worried that the nationalists were losing ground to the Communists. The US provided a moderate amount of aid in the hope that, combined with a lot of self-help by the Nationalists, it would help defeat the Communists. Following the failure of this first attempt, the US wrote off the KMT regime when it retreated to Taiwan. Salvation for the KMT came from the Korean War, as mentioned in Chapter 3, which triggered sudden US interest in defending the island as part of a global effort to contain Communism. The US thereafter extended massive military and economic aid to Taiwan.

Taiwanese authorities actually like to recall the period when they benefited from outside help. They credit aid for the island's amazing economic development and generally have positive views of foreign aid. The first success story of economic assistance to developing countries, US aid to Taiwan was eventually phased out because Taiwan had reached a level of development where economic growth could sustain itself (Jacoby, 1966).

Taiwan's aid mostly corresponds to the criteria of ODA, as nearly all of Taiwan's allies are regarded as developing countries according to the DAC classification (OECD, 2003, 2005). Does peer pressure help explain Taiwan's decision to provide aid to developing countries? One could argue that Taiwan has no peer because of its unique geopolitical situation, but the Taiwanese authorities refer to the efforts of other wealthy countries and implicitly regard them as benchmarks.

The Taiwanese authorities advance two reasons why Taiwan's ratio of ODA to GDP is lower than the OECD average. First, Taiwan's GDP per capita is not yet on par with the OECD average. Second, the island's lack of international status restricts its capacity to provide aid. This is a valid point in the case of economic aid. In particular, the lack of protection for Taiwanese investments has been described as a problem in countries which do not offer guarantees to Taiwanese investors. For humanitarian aid, the diplomatic status of recipients does not officially influence the process. In contrast, Taiwan asks for the repayment of loans in full, in particular for medical infrastructure projects, if a diplomatic ally defects.

Political and economic norms combined

The focus is here on the difficulty for Taiwan to abide by global transparency and accountability standards. Taiwan says disclosing economic and financial aid data may jeopardise some of their expected outcomes.

TaiwanICDF's budget is approved by the Legislative Yuan. TaiwanICDF's annual reports provide detailed descriptions of programmes and activities, and audited accounts. TaiwanICDF does not break amounts down into individual projects or recipient countries. Aid officials say they do not want to see bidding wars between recipients. The amounts of bilateral soft loans to diplomatic allies are also not publicized. There too the stated reason is that Taiwan does not want recipients to start a bidding competition and demand more aid, should such information be made public (interview with Michel Ching-long Lu, 21 September 2004). The government does not want its budgetary planning to be disrupted by such demands.

In one instance, though, the amount of aid provided to a former ally, Senegal, was made public by Chen Shui-bian himself. He argued that 'the cost of the West African nation's move to switch diplomatic recognition to Beijing needed to be made public' (*Straits Times*, 8 November 2005) and stated that Taiwan 'had spent NT$5 billion (US$148.4 million) on assistance programs to Senegal since the time when the African nation switched diplomatic recognition from Beijing to Taipei in 1996' (*China Post*, 8 November 2005). This means Taiwan gave Senegal around US$15 million annually. MoFA officials declined to comment. The disclosure

> drew criticisms that the President himself was undermining Taiwan's diplomacy by breaching the rule that monetary assistance given to the island's allies is to be kept confidential. An opposition lawmaker said Mr Chen might have 'committed an act of revolt or treason' and should be brought to trial.
>
> (*Straits Times*, 8 November 2005)

KMT Legislator John Chiang argued that the disclosure could undermine Taiwan's diplomatic position and referred to 'public concerns that Taiwan's other diplomatic allies might ask for the same level of financial aid as Senegal had received' (*China Post*, 8 November 2005). The disclosure was a surprise as Chen Shui-bian had previously said that he did not want the PRC to know how much aid Taiwan was giving to its allies. It can be argued that the culture of secrecy that started in the KMT years has not yet given way to full democratic openness and disclosure and that, as democracy matures in Taiwan and many of the countries it helps, disclosure and openness will improve.

But it can also be argued that full disclosure will not be possible as long as Taiwan's international status remains in limbo. Can Taiwan afford to disclose all its aid commitments when China does not? Can Taiwan outbid China? The Chinese government is under no internal pressure to disclose aid commitments. Besides, competition from the mainland has been keen in recent years. For example, Dominica, a tiny Caribbean nation with only 70,000 inhabitants, switched back official diplomatic recognition to Beijing in 2004. The PRC reportedly offered the island a US$112 million aid package, representing more than $1,500 for every inhabitant (*New York Times*, 31 March 2004). If this is true, Taiwan cannot afford to compete. Taiwan's budgetary resources are limited, and the democratic oversight process would lead to hard questions by legislators if the MoFA were to request amounts of this magnitude for aid packages.

Conversely, it can be argued that the current policy is unsustainable anyway. Taiwan's pool of allies is steadily shrinking. Massive promises of aid are no longer sufficient to lure prospective targets. When the Republic of China was courting Macedonia in the late 1990s, figures of up to $2 billion were floating around. Such figures were never confirmed by Taiwanese authorities. Then President Lee Teng-hui promised US$300 million for the reconstruction of Kosovo, on condition that the aid be channelled through the UN. The Macedonia episode provided a rare example of the real intentions of the Taiwanese authorities. Pressed by legislators, then Foreign Minister Jason Hu acknowledged that total aid to Macedonia amounted to US$10 million, and that this was the figure the authorities had in mind throughout (Tubilewicz, 2001).

The episode highlighted an even more difficult issue for Taiwan. The tension between political and economic norms is not just about disclosure but also about China's political clout, which Taiwan simply cannot hope to offset with material resources. Just after Macedonia recognized Taiwan, China vetoed the renewal of UNPREDEP, the mission the UN Security Council had sent to the country to help it cope with the Kosovo crisis (United Nations Department of Public Information, 1999). Liberia too switched diplomatic recognition to China to gain China's support for and participation in a UN peacekeeping mission in the aftermath of civil war. The MoFA's spokesman suggested that China's status as a permanent member of the UN Security Council presented Taiwan with yet another problem, as countries seeking a seat on the Council would need China's support.

> Blaming Wade for the break in diplomatic ties between the two countries, Lu said Wade asked Taiwan for more grant money, and turned to Beijing

> for cash after his requests were turned down by Taipei. Considering his nation [Senegal] a big country in Africa, Lu said Wade believes that friendship with Beijing will help his country's pursuit for permanent membership on the UN Security Council.
>
> (*China Post*, 8 November 2005)

The amounts granted by the Department of Health, in particular to Taiwanese NGOs, are not known in detail. The disbursements of loans to allied governments earmarked for the financing of medical aid projects are not reported on a regular basis, and never broken down by recipient. In 2002, publicized medical aid programmes included a US$1 million donation to the Global Fund, one third of US$1 million to CARE-France for the Chad AIDS project and four medical missions estimated at around US$500,000 each.

This means that the combined budget of publicized operations only represented 10 to 15 per cent of Taiwan's total ODA to health. The conclusion here is that transparency, with regard to official humanitarian and medical aid, is only partial and relative. Partial, because it only applies to some of Taiwan's ODA to health and humanitarian contributions. Relative, because the reporting format used by TaiwanICDF does not allow a detailed analysis by project or recipient country.

Taiwanese officials in recent years aggregated figures for aid operations, in particular to Afghanistan and Iraq, carried out under the name 'Love from Taiwan'. In these operations the government took the lead in terms of communications and logistics but failed to provide figures identifying clearly the respective contributions of government agencies, businesses and NGOs.

Taiwan still falls short of the transparency standards established by OECD/DAC. The DAC has elaborated guidelines on a wide range of topics, including aid statistics, aid effectiveness and donor practices, aid untying and governance, and capacity development. While the recommendations of the various working groups are not binding on members, they are made publicly. The reasoning is that this may lead to the adoption of best practices under peer pressure.

Taiwan, under the name Chinese Taipei, is part of a group of emerging, non-DAC donors with which the Development Aid Committee interacts. The DAC has the highest institutional standing of all OECD committees, in particular in terms of level of representation, as it predated the creation of the OECD (Masujima, 2004). DAC took the initiative of a policy dialogue with 'non-OECD governments with significant aid programmes' but 'when updating its outreach strategy recently, the DAC did not single out Chinese Taipei for policy dialogue' (Sedemund, e-mail, 19 August 2008). Taiwan started reporting its aid consistently to the DAC in 2005 'at a very aggregate level, with a breakdown only between multilateral and bilateral aid. There is not a breakdown available between grants, loans and aid in kind' (Sedemund, e-mail, 19 August 2008).

This suggests that Taiwan may not be very eager to open its official assistance to the scrutiny of other official donors. Unlike Korea and the Czech

Republic (other non-DAC donors), Taiwan has not approached the DAC for a review of its aid. Taiwan does not refer specifically to DAC norms but refers selectively to issues discussed by DAC members, in particular tied aid. Taiwan claims that all the aid it provides is untied, as recipients are not obliged to source goods and services from Taiwanese companies.

Governance actors revisited

At first sight the actors involved in Taiwan's aid in general, and medical and humanitarian aid in particular, bear striking resemblance with counterparts elsewhere. Government agencies carry out official aid programmes. Businesses support aid efforts through cash or in-kind donations. Humanitarian NGOs channel volunteers' efforts and individual donations.

But this resemblance is also misleading. Government agencies are not exactly emulating the behaviour of government agencies elsewhere. Businesses are sometimes requested to do more than donating cash or in-kind resources. Finally, NGOs do not enjoy all the freedoms and possibilities that their counterparts in other wealthy, democratic countries enjoy.

State organizations

Although TaiwanICDF is a statutory body, its true nature is open to question. Surprisingly, in one of its brochures the MoFA describes the Fund as an NGO. 'Some NGOs are based on diplomatic considerations, such as the International Cooperation and Development Fund (ICDF) which provides post-disaster emergency relief, as well as medical, sanitary and nutritional assistance in countries maintaining diplomatic relations with Taiwan' (NGO Affairs Committee, 2006: 68). This is surprising because the fund does not focus primarily on emergency relief or medical assistance but on economic aid, which represents the bulk of its activity. In addition, the board of directors, statutorily composed of senior government ministers, heads of government agencies, scholars and industrialists, does not include any NGO representative.

The financial operations of the fund lead to questions about its nature. TaiwanICDF receives a yearly budget line from the Legislative Yuan, listed in TaiwanICDF's statement of income as 'revenues from contracted projects'. To these revenues correspond 'contracted project expenses' of the same amount. This suggests that for these contracted projects ICDF is just the vehicle through which the government carries out certain operations.

Besides contracted projects, TaiwanICDF's statement of income lists seven categories of revenue, including revenues from investment and lending, interest from funds, gain on disposal of investments and foreign exchange gain, and seven categories of expenses, including investment and lending expenses, education and training expenses, technical cooperation expenses, operational and planning expenses and general and administrative expenses. Surprisingly, no budgetary appropriations correspond to the fund's education, training and technical cooperation expenses. Besides, there are also no budgetary appropriations for operational and planning expenses, which include outlays for humanitarian aid, or general and administrative expenses.

In short, TaiwanICDF does not receive any budget in the form of grants. All the money received through budgetary appropriations is earmarked for investments and loans to economic development projects in aid recipient countries (interview with Stephen Lee, 21 September 2004). The amounts granted by TaiwanICDF for education and training, technical cooperation and humanitarian aid are taken from the profits of investment and lending operations. Therefore, and notwithstanding its non-profit status, the business model of TaiwanICDF is closer to that of a development bank with a global corporate philanthropy programme than to that of an official, statutory aid agency.

This leads to the question: what would happen if TaiwanICDF were to turn a loss instead of a profit? TaiwanICDF has so far been able to sustain its granting programme, but there is no institutional guarantee that such a programme could be sustained at all times. As noted in its 2003 annual report, TaiwanICDF is 'a non-profit organization that derives most of its income from interest on long-term lending and short-term investments, which are often influenced by global economic conditions' (TaiwanICDF, 2004: 122). More specifically, it is acknowledged that 'ICDF operations present various latent risks, including risks from bad loans, wrong investment decisions, unfulfilled investment guarantees, and interest rates fluctuations' (TaiwanICDF, 2004: 126).

These are not just theoretical risks, as TaiwanICDF statements of income show. In particular, from 2002 to 2003, interest from fund fell from NT$231 million to NT$171 million, gain on disposal of investments fell from NT$150 million to NT$93 million and foreign exchange gain fell from NT$157 million to NT$90 million. When aggregated, these three sources of income fell 34 per cent year-on-year. This had consequences for the programmes financed from this income. While technical cooperation and operational and planning expenses were nearly unchanged, education and training expenses fell 25 per cent year-on-year (TaiwanICDF, 2004). Besides, in 2006, banking and finance expenses reached NT$176 million, against NT$70 million budgeted, 'due to recognized bad debts, which were higher than anticipated' (TaiwanICDF, 2007: 75). As a result, international human resource development and technical cooperation expenses were cut down to NT$61 million and NT$65 million, respectively, against NT$82 million and NT$86 million budgeted.

Another issue is that TaiwanICDF has no expertise in humanitarian aid. The Fund has a technical cooperation department and an education and training department, but no humanitarian assistance department. Humanitarian assistance programmes are under the responsibility of the Policy, Planning and Programming Department. TaiwanICDF inherited a humanitarian mandate from the International Humanitarian Relief Fund (IHRF) in 1997, but had not yet set up a professionally-staffed department to handle humanitarian programmes as of June 2004 (interview with Stephen Lee, 21 September 2004). This raises questions about TaiwanICDF's capacity to respond to humanitarian emergencies, compounding the long-term uncertainty over funding for humanitarian operations and medical cooperation programmes.

The status of some other actors involved in Taiwan's medical and humanitarian assistance is unclear. In particular, TaiwanICDF reported carrying out three of the ten international humanitarian assistance projects listed in its 2003 Annual Report through such entities: the Taiwan–Tibet Exchange Foundation, the Taiwan–Russia Association and the Taiwan–Mongolia Association. The Taiwan–Tibet Exchange Foundation was described by the Prime Minister of the Tibetan Government-in-exile as a purely non-governmental Taiwanese organization with which the Tibetan Government-in-exile had nothing to do (Friends of Tibet, 2003). Although the Taiwan–Tibet Exchange Foundation claimed to be a non-governmental organization, its Secretary-General, Joseph Wu, was also the deputy secretary-general of the Presidential Office. He described the foundation as 'a quasi-official institution because it receives part of its financial support from the private sector and the rest from the government' (*Taipei Times*, 7 July 2003). He added that

> Its mission is to augment ties between Taiwan and the Tibet government-in-exile. It also serves as the counterpart to the Tibet Religious Foundation of the Dalai Lama, which has operated in Taipei since 1997 as the representative office of the Tibetan government-in-exile.
>
> (*Taipei Times*, 7 July 2003)

Asked whether the foundation would eventually take over the role of the Mongolian and Tibetan Affairs Commission, Wu further elaborated that

> the foundation will serve as an interim agency after the Mongolian and Tibetan Affairs Commission is abolished and before all of the commission's Tibet-related businesses are transferred to the Ministry of Foreign Affairs. It's like the Taiwan Mongolia Exchange Foundation, which still exists after the visa business of the Mongolian and Tibetan Affairs Commission was transferred to the foreign ministry in February last year. If you ask me about the planned abolition of the Mongolian and Tibetan Affairs Commission, I think it makes perfect sense because the organization is not recognised by the Tibetan government-in-exile and has a historic burden.
>
> (*Taipei Times*, 7 July 2003)

The historic burden was further described by him as follows:

> The Tibetan government-in-exile has lost its trust in the Mongolian and Tibetan Affairs Commission, which views Tibet as part of China under the ROC on Taiwan. It is one of the main reasons why the commission's many efforts don't receive much appreciation from the Tibetan government-in-exile in Dharmsala, India, although the commission has earmarked humanitarian aid and other assistance to the Tibetan government-in-exile annually.
>
> (*Taipei Times*, 7 July 2003)

The state organizations Taiwan uses to channel its aid have complex identities. The case of the Taiwan–Tibet Exchange Foundation points to added complexity when dealing with another unrecognized government such as the Tibetan Government-in-exile.

Market organizations

Taiwanese businessmen have been enrolled in aid efforts as donors of cash resources and in-kind contributions, in particular through the 'Love from Taiwan' operations in Afghanistan in 2001, Iraq in 2003 and after the December 2004 Indian Ocean tsunami. While businesses around the world contributed similarly to medical assistance and emergency relief projects, Taiwanese businessmen were sometimes invited to play less conventional roles, as in the case of the polio eradication campaign. Taiwanese businessmen were primarily involved in that campaign though the Rotary Club. Rotary International was the most prominent NGO involved in the campaign in terms of fundraising. The Taiwan chapter was one of the most successful fundraisers of all Rotary clubs worldwide for the polio eradication campaign and the contribution of Taiwan Rotarians was topped up by the Taiwanese government. The contribution of Taiwanese businessmen, combined with that of the government, was widely publicized, and hailed by the government as one of the most outstanding contributions to global health. It has since been listed in many publications by the government in support of the WHO bid.

More recently, Taiwan Rotarians were active in providing relief to people affected by the December 2004 Indian Ocean tsunami, particularly in Indonesia. Another relevant international group is the Kiwanis, often mentioned by Taiwanese aid officials. Although the Kiwanis were founded in the US, the Taiwan chapter is the largest in the world. The Rotary Club and the Kiwanis are not strictly speaking business organizations; they are also open to professionals. But it is interesting that the Taiwanese chapters of both organizations are very active and 'oversized', while Taiwan's status in the global arena is 'undersized'. Is there a link? This is an area for further research.

Taiwanese businessmen were also enrolled in other ways. In particular, as discussed in Chapter 3, overseas Taiwanese businessmen were regarded by Taiwanese diplomats as a prime link to local authorities, in particular in Southeast Asia (Chen, 2002). Taiwanese businessmen were also identified by Taiwanese humanitarian NGOs, first and foremost the Tzu Chi Foundation, as essential links. In particular, the Tzu Chi Foundation realized that Taiwanese businessmen based in Thailand would be key to the long-term sustainability of aid programmes in favour of the Chinese ethnic minorities in Northern Thailand. The internationalization and overseas development of Tzu Chi paralleled Taiwanese emigration (Huang, 2002). The role of Taiwanese businessmen in aid activities, and what is expected from them by both the government and NGOs, goes beyond what can be described as 'ambassadors of goodwill' or 'good global citizens'. This suggests that, in the context of Taiwan, businesses and businessmen's organizations are pushed to do more than what their counterparts elsewhere do.

Civil society organizations

Taiwanese humanitarian NGOs face two sets of constraints. One is derived from the status of non-profit organizations (NPOs) in Taiwan and the other from their involvement in overseas activities. NPOS in Taiwan may register as associations or foundations, but the registration process involves a relatively high degree of discretion by the authorities. The procedures are quite complex and involve a large number of laws and regulations (Feng, 1999). Associations can only raise funds from their members. Humanitarian organizations usually need to raise funds from the public and register as foundations. Foundations have to register with the ministry or government agency responsible for their sector of activity. 'There are thirteen such governing agencies, each with their own regulations governing foundations' (Feng, 1999: 316).

The Ministry of Education supervises the largest number of foundations (587), followed by the National Health Administration and the Ministry of Interior Affairs for foundations in the health and social welfare sectors, respectively (Feng, 1999). But there is no authorized agency under the Ministry of Foreign Affairs where NPOs involved in international affairs or international cooperation could register. This suggests that the institutional environment of Taiwanese civil society organizations involved in international cooperation is a grey area.

One may wonder why this is the case. A convergent view among persons interviewed for this study was that MoFA officials are rather wary of independent-minded civil society activists. The lack of a clear institutional framework for civil society organizations involved in international cooperation may be intentional and provide authorities with easy ways of discouraging activities or co-opting activists, as discussed in Chapter 3. NPOS are not required by law to disclose financial information (Feng, 1999).

Besides legal and statutory requirements, humanitarian NGOs face problems because of Taiwan's geopolitical situation. Activities, programmes or plans may be blocked by the PRC government, suspicious of Taiwanese medical and humanitarian NGOs, or jeopardized by Taiwanese authorities. The following examples illustrate these difficulties.

The Taiwan Roots Medical Peace Corps (TRMPC) experienced difficulties in negotiating access to countries which recognize the PRC. These countries may be reluctant to antagonize China by letting in a few medical volunteers in the country, even for short-term missions. For these reasons, negotiations to obtain visas are usually low-profile. The PRC may otherwise put pressure on its diplomatic allies to deny visas to Taiwanese medical teams planning to visit the country.

In one instance, the TRMPC was forced to cancel a medical mission to Tanzania even after its volunteers had secured visas. The TRMPC failed to obtain the necessary licenses to practice as medical workers in the country, as Beijing put pressure on the Tanzanian government. The TRMPC redirected the mission and sent it to Gambia, one of Taiwan's diplomatic allies (interview with Grace Lee, 23 September 2004). In another example, 'Taipei Overseas Peace

Service, a Taiwan-based NGO mainly working on development in Indochina, cooperated with UNICEF (UN Children's Fund) on an education project in 1998. The collaboration lasted just one year, due to objections from China' (*Taipei Times*, 1 November 2000).

The Taiwanese authorities may also create problems for Taiwanese NGOs. In one instance, the TIMA had planned a workshop on public health in Vietnam with NGOs from various Southeast Asian countries. As Taiwan's Ministry of Foreign Affairs, one of the main sponsors, insisted forcefully on being officially invited to the meeting, the Vietnamese government backed down and the meeting had to be cancelled (interview with Song-lih Huang, 22 September 2004). In another example,

> in order to glean first-hand information about the Chinese health situation, health officials are reported to have asked a Taiwanese organisation to play some kind of 'health spy' role on the Chinese side of the Strait. The organisation preferred to protect its autonomy and to pursue its work in China: it unhesitatingly rejected the proposition.
>
> (Rollet, 2005)

But the most dramatic instance was certainly the cancellation of the medical mission run by Pingtung Christian Hospital in Mzuzu after Malawi broke diplomatic links with Taiwan. The mission, originally run by TaiwanICDF, was handed over to Pingtung Christian Hospital in 2002. MoFA Deputy Minister Yang Tzu-pao was reported as saying that 'all diplomatic affairs – including all Taiwan sponsored humanitarian aid and projects – would cease immediately' (*Taipei Times*, 15 January 2008). Although the medical team wanted to continue their work with AIDS patients, they had to leave. As explained by the team leader, 'Though Pingtung Christian hospital is a non-governmental organization, the Malawi medical team was primarily sponsored by Taiwan government. So, we need to obey the official order' (Chen, e-mail, 28 August 2008).

Humanitarian organizations undertaking projects and programmes overseas may face numerous difficulties in terms of access, in particular in war-torn countries. NGOs may also face pressure from their own government, in particular when they operate in sensitive conflict areas. But the situation of Taiwanese humanitarian NGOs is unique. Not only do they have to deal with the problems all other humanitarian organizations face, they also have to deal with the dual obstacle of China's hostility and Taiwan's isolation. Taiwan's radical isolation and restricted diplomatic space makes China's pressure and hostility very effective. There is hardly any safe area for Taiwanese humanitarian NGOs overseas because nearly all of Taiwan's official diplomatic alliances are precarious and under constant pressure from the PRC. Ironically, mainland China may be the only country where Taiwanese humanitarian organizations face fewer problems than other humanitarian organizations. In particular, it was reported that 'the Ministry of Civil Affairs had formally approved the application by Tzu Chi to establish the charity foundation in China. The new organization is the first foundation chaired by a legal representative who is a non-resident of the mainland' (*China Post*, 28 February 2008).

As mentioned earlier, the Taiwanese Red Cross is officially a branch of the Chinese Red Cross. On its website the Chinese Red Cross lists the Taiwanese Red Cross as one of its 34 provincial branches, which also include the Hong Kong Red Cross and the Macao Red Cross. But the Taiwanese Red Cross is the only provincial branch to which the Chinese Red Cross does not provide any link on its website. In contrast, the Taiwanese Red Cross portrays itself as the Red Cross Society of the Republic of China, created in 1904. Its disputed status makes it difficult for the Taiwanese Red Cross to fulfil its mandate as defined by Red Cross statutes.

Because the International Federation of Red Cross and Red Crescent Societies (IFRC) recognizes the PRC as the only China, its contacts with the Taiwanese Red Cross are institutionally limited and closely scrutinized by the PRC. In particular, the support programmes the Federation develops for the Taiwanese Red Cross are limited in scope (interview with Leif Dierks, 22 September 2004). The dissemination of international humanitarian law is accepted by Beijing but the IFRC is not allowed to support the institutional development of the Taiwanese Red Cross. Meanwhile the Taiwanese Red Cross contributes financially to relief operations overseas, although that support is limited by these institutional constraints.

The attitude of the Taiwanese government towards the Red Cross is somewhat ambivalent. The Taiwanese authorities have often used the Red Cross to channel aid overseas, starting with former Soviet republics in 1991 (Taiwan International Medical Alliance, 2004). But when the Taiwanese Red Cross responded to the Bam earthquake in Iran in 2003, the Taiwanese government chose to channel its contribution through other organizations (interview with Christian Li, 22 September 2004). The reason was probably the political affiliation of the President of the Taiwanese Red Cross with the KMT at a time when the DPP was in power (personal communication from a senior Red Cross executive, 23 October 2004). In the early 1990s the Taiwanese Red Cross played a pioneering role in establishing contacts and fostering confidence-building measures in cross-strait relations. This role is highlighted in the Jinmen Agreement, signed by the Red Cross Societies on both sides of the Taiwan Strait, which focused in particular on the repatriation of illegal immigrants.

Governance processes revisited

The processes of medical aid governance mix vertical approaches with horizontal partnerships. In the 1970s the focus started shifting from vertical eradication strategies to horizontal approaches highlighting primary healthcare and access issues. The trend then seemed to move in the opposite direction. With the Millennium Development Goals, the pendulum appeared to move back halfway, with a mix of horizontal and vertical targets and strategies.

Linking arrangements

Over time institutional arrangements in medical aid processes have become increasingly complex: from the lone, unitary medical actor (WHO) to the involvement of other IGOs (UNICEF, World Bank); from 'sovereign' agencies to multi-agency arrangements, first on a small scale with Tropical Disease Research (TDR), then on a larger scale with UNAIDS; and from governmental or intergovernmental agencies to more inclusive ones, like the Global Fund. As more actors got involved in less hierarchical ways, NGOs moved from the status of 'NGO in official relations' (WHO) to partnership in service delivery (UNICEF) and board membership (UNAIDS). More recently, NGOs' multifaceted partnership with the Global Fund involved board membership, project evaluation and implementation. These evolutions are remarkable as over the period states remained the primary donors. Mirroring what happened in medical aid governance, the responses to humanitarian emergencies also evolved rapidly, as discussed in Chapter 2. In short, both medical aid governance and global disaster response led to increasingly complex processes, as seemingly intractable problems called for innovative solutions. New organizations were created. In the absence of an unquestionable coordinating authority, interaction patterns became increasingly complex as the number of organizations involved rose.

In Taiwan the interactions between the Ministry of Foreign Affairs and the Department of Health were for a long time limited. The creation of TaiwanIHA may be an effort to strengthen the links but the extent of the institutional commitment of the MoFA and the DoH is not clear.

The three main contributions of Taiwan's government – to polio eradication, the Global Fund and UNAIDS – followed three different modus operandi. Taiwan eliminated polio in 1985. In 2000, 'thirty-seven countries in the western Pacific region were declared polio-free by the organization. China was also on the list, and Taiwan was included as a part of China' (*Taipei Times*, 31 October 2000). Taiwan complained that the WHO did not recognize Taiwan's own achievement, independently from China. In the 1990s Taiwan wanted to contribute directly to WHO's polio eradication campaign:

> 'We've donated more than US$1 million through Rotary International to the WHO's worldwide polio eradication program last year,' Hsu [Hsu-mei, deputy director-general at the Center for Disease Control] said. 'Taiwan will donate US$10 million, divided between the government and Rotary International in Taiwan, to WHO in installments over five years.' But health officials noted that Taiwan won't be recognized on the WHO's donor list because the sponsorship was done through Rotary International. The WHO declined to accept Taiwan's donation in the name of Taiwan.
>
> (*Taipei Times*, 31 October 2000)

Rotary International was one of the main partners and major contributors to the campaign, and certainly the most significant non-state actor. Taiwanese authorities capitalized on the momentum created by a non-state actor and gained approval, recognition and visibility on the way.

Taiwanese aid officials since failed to replicate this success in part because they did not keep up with the rapidly evolving medical aid scene. In particular, they were slow to internalize the dynamics of the Millennium Declaration and the Millennium Development Goals, which is radically different from the eradication paradigm. Taiwanese authorities did not involve civil society organizations in their contribution to the Global Fund. The MoFA disburses and oversees Taiwan's contribution to the Global Fund, listed as a contribution from the Health Authorities of Taiwan on the website of the Global Fund (Global Fund, 2006a).

The personal connection between the former Minister of Health of Taiwan and former US Secretary for Health Tommy Thompson appears to be an important reason why Taiwan contributed twice to the Global Fund (interview with Peter Chang, 9 June 2004). The official contribution was not matched by private contributions and its visibility was low. This is ironic as it all happened under Chen Shui-bian's administration, who advocated people's diplomacy and civil society involvement. How can we make sense of this?

In the case of the polio eradication campaign, Taiwanese authorities did not see the channelling of their contribution through Taiwan's Rotary Club and Rotary International as the best solution, as it was not listed as such. Nevertheless, they saw an opportunity to demonstrate both Taiwan's commitment to a global public good (the eradication of a disease) and the restrictions that Taiwan's status placed on a more significant contribution. In contrast, in the case of Taiwan's official donation to the Global Fund to fight AIDS, tuberculosis and malaria, Department of Health Head Lee Ming-liang was clearly satisfied that the donation could be made under the name 'Taiwan':

> 'That means, when we make the donation, the receipt would clearly state that the money comes from Taiwan,' Lee said during a press conference after his meeting with [US Secretary for Health Tommy] Thompson at the Intercontinental Hotel in Geneva. 'We could have made the donation through some private channels, such as under the name of the Foundation of Medical Professionals Alliance in Taiwan, or in my private capacity, but that's the wrong approach,' Lee said. 'Since the donation comes from taxpayers' money, I find it necessary to state clearly that the donation comes from Taiwan,' Lee said.
>
> (*Taipei Times*, 16 May 2002)

Taiwan's official contribution to the regional UNAIDS prevention project in Chad is yet another case. In this instance, the Taiwanese government channelled its donation through the French branch of an international humanitarian organization, CARE-France. Without the personal connection between the CEO of CARE-France and the Head of overseas relief operations of the Tzu Chi Foundation, it is unlikely that CARE-France would have received this grant from the MoFA (interview with Hsiang-Ming Hsu, 24 September 2004). The initial plan involved a significant input from Taiwan in terms of human resources, which never materialized. Although the feasibility study was carried out jointly by CARE-France and the Ministry of Foreign Affairs, TaiwanICDF thereafter failed to find a Taiwanese French-speaking doctor to work from N'Djamena on the project. Taiwan's contribution, though far from insignificant, remained only financial.

The contributions to both the Global Fund and the Chad projects were managed by the MoFA, with little input from the Department of Health and hardly any from Taiwanese civil society organizations. While the operations mentioned above are among the most visible, they only represent a small fraction of Taiwan's ODA to health and official contributions to humanitarian operations. Other operations include the medical missions, humanitarian assistance and soft loans for infrastructure projects. The processes relevant to these various operations are diverse.

The medical missions are usually directly managed, manned and supervised by TaiwanICDF but in 2002 Pingtung Christian Hospital was given the task to 'take over responsibility for the Malawi Medical Mission. This is the only medical mission funded by the government to be operated by a hospital' (*Liberty Times*, 27 October 2004). As Malawi broke diplomatic relations with Taiwan in January 2008, the mission was cancelled.

The collaboration between state and non-state actors in Taiwan's medical cooperation now includes short-term mobile medical missions run by TaiwanICDF in partnership with Taiwanese hospitals and medical schools. These missions also target countries which are not necessarily diplomatic allies. As noted by TaiwanICDF's Chen Chi-fu,

> the quality medical services that missions provide are not something that China can beat merely by spending money. 'If diplomacy is like a tree, medical missions are like the roots which nurture the tree, make it grow and bear the fruit of friendship and respect,' he says. 'We've put down deep roots.'
>
> (*Taiwan Review*, 30 November 2006)

The contribution to the Global Fund and the Chad UNAIDS project were significant because they were publicly discussed and specifically approved by the Legislative Yuan. But the fact that both projects were initiated on the basis of personal connections also points to a lack of policy direction. True, larger amounts were contributed by the government to other medical aid projects, including soft loans for medical infrastructure projects but the amounts, terms and use of those loans are not open to public scrutiny.

In response to overseas emergencies the Taiwanese authorities pushed for increased cooperation between state and non-state actors, at least in terms of logistics and communication. It is also not clear how far Taiwanese aid organizations coordinate with others in such cases, as Taiwan remains a non-entity for UN relief organizations, including the UNHCR, UNICEF and the WFP. The only area where Taiwan has made some progress is information sharing. Tzu Chi was the first Taiwanese organization to report on its disaster relief activities on Reliefweb, UNOCHA's website and has done so on several occasions. Taiwan's government followed suit in the aftermath of the 2004 Indian Ocean tsunami.

The operating modes of Taiwan's humanitarian and medical aid organizations are very diverse, in particular in terms of the partnerships they establish. Government organizations involved in official assistance (MoFA, TaiwanICDF, DoH, CoA) display a great diversity of linking arrangements, but weak linkages between them. Linking arrangements seem to be driven by personal contacts or communication and public relations needs more than policy. On the NGO side, Tzu Chi has its own operating model and network and appears to enjoy a wider array of linkages and partnerships than Taiwan's government itself. This is a reflection of the low status of Taiwan among state actors and of Tzu Chi's achievements in humanitarian and medical aid overseas.

Policy instruments

The physical instruments used by the government include the rescue unit of the Taipei Fire Brigade, airlifting operations and visa facilitation for NGO volunteers and staff. However, airlifting is carried out by Taiwan's airlines, not government airplanes, and visas can only be obtained for countries where Taiwan has official or unofficial diplomatic representations. Elsewhere, NGOs rely on expatriate Taiwanese businessmen's networks (interview with Grace Lee, 23 September 2004). Taiwan's status restricts its ability to use physical instruments. For instance Taiwan cannot use its Navy for overseas disaster relief.

Material instruments include grants, loans and aid-in-kind. In 1978 the DAC advised that 'members should endeavour fully to maintain or achieve as soon as possible an average grant element in their ODA commitments of at least 86 per cent' (OECD, 1978). Furthermore, the DAC clarified in a working paper that humanitarian assistance is not counted as ODA (OECD, 2004) but debt cancellation and forgiveness were accepted as ODA instruments. Loans qualify as aid if there is a concessional element of at least 25 per cent when compared to a reference interest rate of 10 per cent per annum (OECD, 2001).

Loans make sense for economic development projects which offer clear returns on investments. The rationale is less compelling for social infrastructure projects such as schools or medical facilities. The pay-back horizon is distant and difficult to assess on a project basis, due to the multidimensional links between education, health and economic growth. In addition, overemphasis on cost recovery for healthcare services was shown to result in significant lower take-up (Whitehead *et al.*, 2001).

Taiwan's medical aid consists mostly of bilateral soft loans extended to allies for medical infrastructure, like the hospital built by Taiwan in Mzuzu, Malawi at a cost of US$18 million (*Central News Agency*, 7 July 2002). Do these loans qualify as ODA in the sense accepted by OECD donors? This cannot be ascertained as the terms are not publicized.

Government funding for Taiwanese NGOs is scarce. Aid officials would apparently like to do more. While some NGOs accept some funding from the government, they also appear eager to limit it to retain their independence (interview with Grace Lee, 23 September 2004). Besides, Tzu Chi does not solicit funds from the government. While NGOs everywhere must balance government funding and independence, Taiwan's status and the dual pressure from both the Taiwanese government and the PRC on Taiwanese NGOs may exacerbate the dilemma. NGOs in other donor countries may not always see this clearly, especially when governments portray themselves as standard-bearers of human rights or humanitarian values, but NGOs in Taiwan appear to be acutely aware of the consequences of accepting government funding.

The government uses symbolic instruments intensively and in particular capitalizes on aid efforts by non-state actors. Taiwanese authorities report all the good deeds carried out by Taiwanese NGOs in print and on their websites. They regularly highlight the contributions of private organizations and portray them as contributions from Taiwan, even when the government plays no operational role. In an example of co-optation, organizations seeking funding from the government to travel to Bangkok for an AIDS conference were granted support on the condition that they join the 'Alliance of Taiwanese NGOs fighting against HIV/AIDS' (Rollet, 2005).

Taiwanese authorities started reporting all aid from the island, including government and private aid, under the labels 'Love from Taiwan' for operations in Afghanistan and Iraq and 'TaiwanIHA' in the aftermath of the 2004 Indian Ocean tsunami. Taiwan's government has a relatively limited range of instruments at its disposal, when compared to other states, and appears to use them in a rather blunt manner towards both other states and non-state actors.

Governance outputs and outcomes revisited

Aid outputs

Bilateral cooperation is often driven by the need for visibility. In the medical field bilateral aid was often criticized for overinvesting in visible structures and equipment, such as hospitals in state or regional capital cities. In contrast, recurrent expenses, such as medical staff salaries and maintenance, were neglected. The WHO repeatedly drew the attention of donors to this problem (WHO, 2000b).

While total ODA by OECD countries more than doubled since the Millennium Summit, from US$50 billion to more than US$100 billion a year, the UN stated that it was 'still far short of estimated needs' and that 'the aid increase is not as impressive as it might appear, taking into account the falling value of the US dollar, in which ODA is measured, and the effects of inflation' (United Nations, 2005). Noting the fall in ODA from 2005 to 2007, the OECD attributed it to 'the end of exceptionally high levels of debt relief (notably for Iraq and Nigeria)' and highlighted that in 2007 'excluding debt relief grants, DAC members' net ODA rose by 2.4%' (OECD, 2008b). Taking stock of these figures, OECD noted that

> At the Gleneagles G8 and UN Millennium +5 summits in 2005, donors committed to increase their aid. The pledges made at these summits, combined with other commitments, implied lifting aid from US$ 80 billion in 2004 to US$ 130 billion in 2010 (at constant 2004 prices). While a few countries have slightly reduced their targets since 2005, the majority of these commitments remain in force.
>
> (OECD, 2008b)

OECD concluded that 'overall, most donors are not on track to meet their stated commitments to scale up aid; they will need to make unprecedented increases to meet their 2010 targets' (OECD, 2008b). As the UN reminded wealthy countries that they should give 0.7 per cent of GDP as ODA, several OECD donors pledged to reach this target or otherwise increase their ODA in a given time frame. Taiwan's ODA amounted to US$514 million in 2007, or 0.13 per cent of GNI. Taiwan's ODA to GNI ratio is below the OECD average of 0.28 per cent (OECD, 2008a).

In recent years DAC members increased ODA to health both in absolute and relative terms. Taiwan's ODA to health ranged from US$19 million to US$28 million yearly from 1998 to 2002 (see Table 6.3) but data are available for recent years.

It could also be argued that the aid budgets of state and non-state actors should be aggregated and regarded as Taiwan's total aid, even when NGOs and the government run their projects independently from each other. This was the US approach after the 2004 Indian Ocean tsunami. Adding up private donations to the US official contribution, the administration fought back those who criticized its stinginess.

Taiwan does not usually aggregate government and private aid data per recipient country but figures were provided for specific operations, such as the polio campaign. The government reportedly gave US$17 million to help Afghan refugees, but it is not clear over what period (Fanchiang, 11 April 2003). TaiwanIHA reported that in the aftermath of the December 2004 Indian Ocean tsunami 'nearly US$200 million of government and private sector funds' were donated (TaiwanIHA, 2007a), which actually included US$50 million from the government and US$150 million from the public to NGOs.

Medical cooperation programmes started in 1962 when Taiwan sent a team to Libya. Some medical volunteers on overseas assignments returned to Taiwan with negative views of their experiences. As a consequence, non-Taiwanese doctors were also recruited for medical missions (telephone interview with Yan-di Chang, 25 October 2004). Possibly to make up for the shortage of candidates or to enhance the people's diplomacy rationale, TaiwanICDF handed over the Malawi medical mission to Pingtung Christian Hospital.

The outputs of the medical missions run by TaiwanICDF ranged from unspecified knowledge and technology transfers in Burkina-Faso to support to surgical and gynaecological departments in Chad, and medical technology services and new management practices in São Tomé and Príncipe, along with a malaria project. The overall amount of medical aid provided by Taiwan is limited. Spreading it over so many different fields makes it more difficult to establish an area of expertise and strengthen impact and visibility. Taiwan's malaria control project in São Tomé and Príncipe provides an illustration of these difficulties.

The dimensions of the archipelago of São Tomé and Príncipe are modest (1,001 sq km) and its population limited (193,000) (Central Intelligence Agency, 2006b). On a mission to São Tomé and Príncipe an expert noted that the archipelago's small size 'and its distance from the African mainland make it amenable for an effective malaria control program' (Teklehaimanot, 2003). He also noted that

> A number of partners such as the UN agencies (WHO & UNICEF), bilateral development organizations (Republic of Taiwan, USAID, Portuguese Research Centers) and the private sector are involved in malaria control and operational research. The input of the Taiwanese group is the most sustentative.
>
> (Teklehaimanot, 2003: 5)

Interestingly, Lay Seng Yung, Secretary of the Taiwan's Embassy in the country, was listed as a technical adviser and member of the Country Coordinating Mechanism set up by the Global Fund (Global Fund, 2006c). But while Taiwan rightly points to its own success in fighting malaria at home, there is no clear evidence that lessons from the Taiwanese experience have been applied in this case.

> By using environmentally friendly insecticide to kill the flies [*sic*] spreading malaria and providing treatment for patients already infected, the mission progressively brought under control the spread of malaria in the country. Similar efforts of the World Health Organization in Africa have remained fruitless, which makes the model of the Taiwan medical mission quite remarkable.
>
> (NGO Affairs Committee, 2006: 76)

This is certainly a big claim. More soberly, UNICEF notes on its website that there is still a long way to go and that

> The threat is even greater in the rainy season, when 464 of every 10,000 people in São Tomé and Príncipe catch malaria, resulting in a 14.8 per cent mortality rate. Yet almost half of all children under the age of five here sleep without an insecticide-treated mosquito bed net.
>
> (UNICEF, 2006b)

Besides, the so-called Taiwan model was tried in São Tomé and Príncipe long before official diplomatic links were established in 1997.

> Past intervention efforts with indoor residual spraying between 1980 and 1983 have demonstrated the technical feasibility of malaria elimination from the island. After three cycles of indoor spraying, mortality was brought down to zero and morbidity level was drastically reduced. However, the program activities were not maintained and resulted in the incidence of malaria and mortality rate bouncing back to epidemic proportions. Thus, while it is technically feasible to drastically reduce malaria in the island, the challenge is the issue of sustainability due to premature withdrawal of control activities.
>
> (Teklehaimanot, 2003: 7)

While the programme of three cycles of indoor spraying conducted by the Taiwanese medical mission to São Tomé and Príncipe, started in 2004, was found effective (Lien *et al.*, 2008), it remains to be seen how sustainable Taiwan's efforts will be in this case. In 2007 TaiwanICDF reported that it held 'a specialized workshop on malaria surveillance in São Tomé and Príncipe' and 'dispatched experts to various countries for short periods to provide on-site training. For instance, Taiwanese experts in the field of malaria prevention were sent to São Tomé and Príncipe' (TaiwanICDF, 2008: 65).

More generally, there is no agreement between the various actors on Taiwan's specific strengths and expertise. AIDS is mentioned by the MoFA as a strong point but the claim was questioned by the Deputy-Director of TaiwanICDF (interview with Stephen Lee, 21 September 2004). In contrast, he highlighted Taiwan's contribution to the fight against TB, but the only project TaiwanICDF lists in this field is 'a community tuberculosis (TB) care project in the Altai region of Russia with the Taiwan-Russia Association' (TaiwanICDF, 2004: 16). The opinion of the Department of Health on this issue is unclear.

On the basis of reports and publications in medical journals, it is suggested here that the work of the medical mission in Malawi was Taiwan's most substantial contribution to medical cooperation. The mission worked from the hospital built in Mzuzu with official Taiwanese assistance. It was noted that

> the hospital is responsible for providing 40 per cent of the city's primary in-hospital health care services and its HIV/Aids program benefits 7,900 patients with ARVs in the city. The program extends to over 70 local clinics in the region with a reach of over 50,000 patients accessing the services
>
> (*Nyasa Times*, 22 January 2008)

In addition, the work of the mission led to publications in medical journals including the *Bulletin of the World Health Organization* (Yu *et al.*, 2005, 2007, 2008).

Taiwan's contribution to multilateral efforts in medical aid appears to be declining in relative terms. Taiwan was the thirteenth largest bilateral donor to the polio campaign for the period 1985–2002 (Global Polio Eradication Initiative, 2006a), but only the twenty-ninth for its contribution to the Global Fund (Global Fund, 2006b).

Taiwan's response to the refugee crisis in Macedonia in 1999 was a sore reminder of Taiwan's isolation. Although Taiwan was reportedly the first country to officially disburse aid to Macedonia and sent a sizeable team to help look after refugees from Kosovo, Taiwan's contribution was hardly noticed, even by close observers (interview with Hervé Caiveau, 13 June 2004). The UNHCR map of the Stenkovac refugee camp where Taiwan's medical team was reportedly deployed, as one would expect, bears no mention of a Taiwanese presence. In a recent publication the government stated that the medical team consisted of TRMPC volunteers and claimed that they 'provided comprehensive care for approximately 40,000 refugees' (Taiwan International Health Action, 2007b: 26). The claim could not be verified independently.

The aid outputs of Taiwanese NGOs also appear to be affected by a lack of clear policies. For instance, there seems to be little interaction between the short-term missions run by the Taiwan Roots Medical Peace Corps and the public health structures in the countries where they intervene. It is only stated that patients who need follow-up will be referred to the local public health structures (interview with Grace Lee, 23 September 2004). Leading international NGOs in the field of medical cooperation have phased out this type of short-term mission involving many foreign volunteers, except in crisis and emergency situations, as they do not result in sustainable outcomes.

Tzu Chi has a clear focus and delivery system. The relevance and added value of its worldwide network was evident in the response of the organization to Hurricane Mitch. Tzu Chi teams based in the US were first on the ground, as it takes a lot more time to fly in from Taiwan to Central America. On this occasion, the Tzu Chi branch in Houston took on the coordination role, even though it was not the most experienced in the US, because it had the best knowledge of Latin America (interview with Hsiang-Ming Hsu, 24 September 2004).

Beyond the narratives provided by NGOs involved in overseas medical or humanitarian aid, it is difficult to provide a reasoned analysis of their outputs and outcomes, as there is an overall lack of financial transparency, standardized data and impact indicators. It is not clear whether NGOs conduct internal evaluations of aid programmes or mandate external evaluations. No specific data could be gathered in this regard.

Measuring aid outputs

Measuring aid outputs can be tricky, as discussed earlier. The OECD/DAC gave a lot of thought to the definition of ODA. While the OECD decided to count debt relief as aid, the UN expressed 'skepticism because the debt relief and humanitarian components have been increasing as a proportion of overall aid, but do not contribute directly to long-term development needs' (United Nations, 2005).

Following the 2004 Indian Ocean tsunami, it was reported 'that Taiwan's government had "decided to boost its aid offer from US$5 million to US$50 million, including US$20 million worth of rice, US$15 million worth of medical supplies and US$15 million in community and harbor reconstruction"' (*Asia Pulse*, 3 January 2005). In the absence of details about the assistance offered, the statement raises output measurement issues.

An issue specific to medical aid is uncertainty over the safeguards included in the TRIPS agreement. Treaty clauses allow countries to resort to compulsory licenses or parallel imports of patented drugs in a public health emergency. This commitment was reaffirmed at the WTO Ministerial Conference in Doha in 2001, but behind-the-scenes arms-twisting in bilateral trade negotiations pushed a number of LDCs to abstain from inserting these safeguards in their respective intellectual property legislations.

Aggregating outputs in monetary terms does not make sense if some programmes use generic drugs while others use patented drugs valued at very different prices. In particular, the World Bank reported establishing a partnership with various institutions including UNICEF, the Global Fund and the Clinton Foundation to help developing countries purchase AIDS medications at lower prices, with savings in the range of US$150–US$400 per patient per year (World Bank, 2004). Since then, prices have been reduced further.

Food aid also raises measurement issues. Like most countries, Taiwan has a long history of protecting its farmers, in particular paddy growers, from cheap imports. The global rice market is rather limited, although some developing countries, notably Thailand and Pakistan, have become significant exporters. Agricultural products were first included in the agenda of multilateral trade negotiations during the Uruguay Round. To enter the WTO Taiwan agreed to open up its rice market to a level of 8 per cent of the Taiwanese consumption, i.e. 144,720 tons per year (S. Huang, 2001). The Taiwanese government simultaneously decided to establish a food aid programme with an allocation of 100,000 tons of rice a year, which offset the impact of WTO accession for Taiwanese paddy growers. The programme raises two issues. Does such a programme qualify as official assistance? How should the output be valued?

According to OECD/DAC norms, food aid should only be counted as official assistance when extended bilaterally and sold on local markets. Cash receipts are then counted as ODA. It can be argued that food aid distributed in other ways, such as food-for-work programmes, also constitutes a resource for the recipient country that would otherwise not be available.

Critics see food aid as a disincentive to local production. Other factors including inadequate agricultural policies, high taxation of farmers, weak enforcement of property or tenancy rights, and law and order have also been shown to impact food production negatively.

One could also argue that Taiwan's rice donations should not qualify as official assistance because the scheme would not have been set up if Taiwan had not joined the WTO. The reasoning would be that Taiwan's rice donations are essentially subsidies to its own rice farmers. The argument is not very convincing. The costs of globalization are internalized in different ways across countries. Countries with a competitive advantage in manufacturing and limited land resources tend to protect their farmers from imports, whereas countries richly endowed in factors of agricultural production such as Australia, Brazil or Canada advocate free trade in commodities on the basis of their own competitive advantage. Blaming Taiwan for its specific location on the international political economy map would not be fair.

Valuation is another issue. Typically, food aid is valued at world prices, as it should be valued at replacement cost from other sources. In the case of Taiwan there was a very large difference between world price and local price. For example, in 2000,

> the guaranteed [farm procurement] price was $981 per ton (japonica rice, milled basis) ... while the average f.o.b. price for Taiwan's rice exports was $144 per ton. Taiwan has exported an average of 100,000 tons of old crop rice from the authorities' central stocks annually over the past 3 years, mostly to African countries that have diplomatic ties with Taiwan.
>
> (S. Huang, 2001: 35)

On what basis is Taiwan's food aid valued? Former Vice Premier Yeh Chu-lan stated that Taiwan's government decided to offer, as part of its aid package to countries affected by the December 2004 Indian Ocean tsunami, 'US$20 million worth of rice' (*Asia Pulse*, 3 January 2005). Valued at 2004 world prices, this would represent nearly the whole yearly quota of 100,000 tons the government gives as food aid. But valued at Taiwan's internal farm procurement prices, this would only represent around 20,000 tons. Similarly, when the Spokesman of the Ministry of Foreign Affairs valued the 4,000 tonnes of rice sent to Jordan in 2003 at US$4 million, he implicitly used domestic prices of around US$1,000 per ton (*Taipei Times*, 24 February 2005).

Outcomes

Linking outputs to outcomes is difficult throughout the entire aid system. As the number and diversity of the actors involved increases, mandates overlap, new paradigms emerge and new governance arrangements are set up, it is not easy to credit any actor or group of actors with a specific achievement. Political will is a key issue and the UN General Assembly staked its credibility on the Millennium Declaration and the MDGs. Funding is also crucial and members of the Development Assistance Committee of the OECD made public pledges. The Millennium Development Goals are an important milestone: a consensus on the outcomes that should be sought in priority, with clear targets set.

Reaching any target of the Millennium Development Goals requires prioritization. What is the most effective combination of outputs to reach a specific outcome? For instance, how best to halt the spread of HIV/AIDS? Clearly, some improvements have taken place. More AIDS patients are treated with ARVs than ever before. But to reach the target, should more resources be allocated to health education, to treatment or to R&D for a vaccine? Should more attention be paid to research and development targeted at the infectious diseases, or to the 'last mile' or 'close-to-client' segment of the healthcare system? (WHO, 2002d; OECD/WHO/DAC, 2003)

One risk is that only those interventions with a proven utility will be regarded as worth underwriting, or legitimately call for a transfer of resources from developed countries to developing ones. A global public good for health, it was suggested, is one that benefits more than one region/continent (Woodward and Smith, 2003). Surprisingly, the same authors argue that, although malaria affects hundreds of millions of people in Africa and Asia and kills over one million each year, it fails to qualify as a global disease as cross-border transmission is low. One wonders if to obtain the label of a truly global disease, an infection has to threaten rich people seriously. In contrast, earlier research on global goods for public health was clearly premised on health as a universal right and not a strictly utilitarian concept (Kaul *et al.*, 1999).

A utilitarian approach to governance would not lead to the same outcomes as one based on rights. If the rationale is to maximize Global Public Goods for Health (GPGHs), the main beneficiaries will likely be patients in large developing countries affected by diseases also prevalent in the developed world, such as TB or AIDS. This is because large developing countries such as Brazil, India or China can better withstand pressure from developed countries, have a strong manufacturing base for generic drugs and benefit from significant economies of scale, and because there are market incentives for pharmaceutical companies to invest in the development of new TB and AIDS drugs.

In contrast, there is hardly any market incentive to invest in R&D for new malaria drugs, and none for most neglected diseases such as leishmaniasis or sleeping sickness. Leishmaniasis patients or African children decimated by malaria are therefore less likely to benefit from the maximization of Global Public Goods for Health, if maximization is understood in utilitarian terms. The lack of market incentives to invest in treatments and cures for neglected diseases and the difficulty for small, poor countries to resist pressure from Western countries and take advantage of the safeguard clauses included in the TRIPS agreement could then impact the attainment of the Millennium Development Goals negatively.

It is too early to say whether the combination of innovative partnerships, increased resources and the scaling-up of interventions with proven positive externalities will make a lasting difference in reducing the global burden of infectious diseases. In spite of the strengthened commitment of the international community to a clear set of targets, it is too early to conclude that the governance systems they have established will deliver.

Taiwan's aid outcomes

It is of course impossible here to carry out an evaluation of Taiwan's aid. Taiwan does not seem eager to see this task fulfilled anyway, and provides few relevant data. What is attempted here is just to provide a few markers regarding the economic impact, human indicators and diplomatic outcomes of Taiwan's aid, whether carried out multilaterally, bilaterally, by NGOs or jointly.

At the macroeconomic level, it is impossible to say whether Taiwan's bilateral aid in general makes a difference. There are many factors involved, and many other providers of aid. The times are gone when a case study of the impact of bilateral aid on development could be neatly delineated, as in the case of US aid to Taiwan in the 1950s and 1960s (Jacoby, 1966). The difference is that there was at the time only one, massive and single-minded provider of aid. Case studies of recipient countries, where aid is significant compared to GDP and Taiwan is a major donor, might help give clearer answers. Taiwan says it focuses on the effectiveness of economic aid, the main component of its aid efforts. In particular, TaiwanICDF is eager to ensure economic aid projects are carried out efficiently. Taiwan's aid is more easily traced when channelled through multilateral organizations. It is more difficult to assess the outcomes of Taiwan's bilateral aid, even though TaiwanICDF claims to follow the World Bank project cycle. Evaluation applies more to economic development projects than to TaiwanICDF's medical and humanitarian projects.

An important issue is that Taiwan has a limited ability to channel contributions in terms of medical aid through multilateral organizations and an even more limited ability to do so with regard to disaster response. Like the WHO, the UNHCR specifically refuses contributions from any organization, state or non-state, associated with Taiwan (interview with Pierre-Bernard Lebas, 9 June 2004).

With regard to human development and relevant indicators including the Human Development Index (HDI) or the health status of beneficiaries, it would be hard to assess the impact of Taiwan's medical and humanitarian aid, as its overall amount remains modest and it is scattered over many fields of activity. While TaiwanICDF emphasizes MDGs and discusses how poverty reduction and healthcare are intertwined, no relevant indicators are provided for TaiwanICDF's contribution. Besides, many factors and other donors are involved. All that can be ascertained is that Taiwan's allies (barring the Vatican) and aid recipients are developing countries, with the vast majority of them categorized as Least Developed Countries (LDCs) or other Low-Income Countries (LICs) (OECD, 2003). Limiting the impact even further, medical cooperation is stopped if a recipient country breaks diplomatic links with Taiwan. As an example, the number of medical missions fell from four to two as Chad defected in 2006 and Malawi in 2008.

Diplomatic outcomes are also difficult to assess. Until Ma's election, Taiwan sought to increase the number of official diplomatic allies. There is no evidence that the provision of medical or humanitarian aid ever pushed any country to switch recognition from Beijing to Taipei. The provision of humanitarian aid may be intended, at least in part, to help cement diplomatic alliances. This was in particular acknowledged in the case of Taiwan's support to the AIDS project run by CARE-France in Chad (*Agence France-Presse*, 12 November 2001). But Chad, which recognized the Republic of China in 1997, defected and switched official diplomatic recognition back to Beijing in August 2006. Taiwan's official humanitarian and medical assistance ranged from US$20 million to US$30 million per year between 1998 and 2002, while total ODA was in the range of

US$300 million per year in the same period. It would therefore be very difficult to ascertain the specific impact of medical and humanitarian aid on any diplomatic switch. Overall aid pledges may have helped, as was the case with Macedonia in 1999. In this instance, the aid package pledged also included aid deemed humanitarian, first for refugees from Kosovo in Macedonia, then for the reconstruction of Kosovo itself. Conversely, there is also no evidence that failure to provide medical or humanitarian aid ever led any of Taiwan's diplomatic allies to withdraw official recognition, even though dissatisfaction with the overall volume of aid was in several instances reported as a reason for Taiwan's aid recipients to switch diplomatic recognition back to China.

The visibility of its contributions may help Taiwan improve its global image and indirectly diplomatic outcomes. In this regard it is interesting to contrast the contribution to the polio campaign and the contribution to the Global Fund. Why did the US$2 million Taiwan government's contribution to the polio campaign go such a long way, while a donation of the same amount to the Global Fund failed to make a similar impression? There are essentially two reasons. First, Taiwan's total contribution to polio eradication was much larger. Including private donations channelled by the Rotary Club, it exceeded US$9 million. Second, the stakes have been considerably raised in the past few years with regard to global health challenges.

The eradication paradigm was relatively inexpensive. The annual cost of the polio eradication campaign peaked at US$700 million in 2005 and was expected to fall below US$200 million by 2008 (Global Polio Eradication Initiative, 2006b). In contrast, 'the Commission on Macroeconomic and Health argues that total needs for donor grants for country level programmes are US$22bn per year by 2007 and US$31bn by 2015 for the least-developed, low- and middle-income countries' (WHO/CMH Support Unit, 2003: 19). Many donor countries, in particular members of the Development Aid Committee of the OECD, have responded at least in part to the challenge and significantly increased their ODA to health. Taiwan's government has not. As Taiwan has not involved non-state actors in its interactions with the Global Fund, its contribution is marginal and lacks visibility.

The comparison between the two operations points to a difference between internal and external visibility. In the case of the polio donation, the target may have been both external and internal. As Taiwan tried to impress the world, issues of protocol and status were not overriding. In the case of the donation to the Global Fund, the primary audience may have been domestic, and the Taiwanese authorities did not care that the world did not notice. The most important point was that domestic constituencies had to be satisfied that Taiwan's status was maintained. Besides, as the contributions to both the Global Fund and the Chad projects were managed by the MoFA with little input from either the Department of Health or Taiwanese civil society organizations, Taiwan's visibility was certainly not maximized.

Taiwan may also have more than one objective in mind, as was the case with the medical mission in Malawi:

> The Taiwan Medical Mission in Malawi, operated by the Pingdong Christian Hospital, has won a nod of approval for their efforts by the people and government of Malawi. Members of the mission this year were able to enter the annual conference of the World Health Organization for the first time in the capacity of being advisors to Malawi. In this instance, Taiwan has been able to chalk up a small victory in its constant diplomatic battle ... The Ministry of Foreign Affairs in recent years has aggressively promoted the use of medical mission as a means of promoting substantive diplomatic work.
>
> (*Liberty Times*, 27 October 2004)

There is certainly a clearer link between Taiwan's medical and humanitarian aid and Taiwan's WHO bid, as stated by the MoFA's former spokesman (interview with Michel Ching-long Lu, 21 September 2004). Unfortunately, the Malawi fiasco epitomizes Taiwan's dilemmas and raises hard questions about its official medical and humanitarian assistance. The Malawi medical mission was the most significant medical cooperation project run by Taiwan. The medical team of 20 expatriates added significant manpower, not to mention funding, skills and equipment, to the provision of healthcare in Northern Malawi. A total of 7,900 AIDS patients were under ARV treatment and the programme benefited up to 50,000 patients through its 70 outreach clinics. One observer assessed that 'Malawi's recent severance of diplomatic ties with Taiwan will have devastating effects on the people of northern Malawi as government does not have contingency plans on the management of essential services' (*Nyasa Times*, 22 January 2008). The impact may never be measured. Sadly, the Taiwanese team, which painstakingly researched issues of treatment discontinuity, compliance and patients transferring out in Northern Malawi, has left.

Clearly, Taiwan was upset by Malawi's defection after 42 years of uninterrupted diplomatic relations, but the MoFA's decision to close the medical mission shows little concern for the patients. Does the MoFA's decision indicate a hardening of Taiwan's policy? Under Taiwan's earlier policy, outstanding loans for medical infrastructure would have been due, but humanitarian assistance would have continued (interview with Stephen Lee, 21 September 2004). With this single decision, the MoFA weakened a key argument of the WHO campaign – that medical and humanitarian issues should not be subordinated to political considerations; Taiwan lost the moral high ground it claimed to hold; and Taiwan exposed as hollow the claim that it could help more if made an observer at the WHO. The cancellation of the medical mission in Malawi had nothing to do with the WHO but was linked to Taiwan's diplomatic fight with China. Thanks to Malawi, a Taiwanese doctor was made a delegate at the World Health Assembly and research by the Taiwan's medical team in Malawi led to work published in the *Bulletin of the World Health Organization*. The decision to scrap its medical mission in the country may lead Taiwan further away from the WHO and appears to be inconsistent with its stated objective. It also leads one to wonder what exactly the MoFA means by 'medical diplomacy'.

Another aspect of the new 'people's diplomacy' defended by Chen Shui-bian was the emphasis on Taiwanese NGOs making their way to the UN. As mentioned in Chapter 6, Tzu Chi was recognized in December 2003 by the United Nation's Department of Public Information (DPI) as an NGO with a significant information programme. Tzu Chi welcomed the move. But although Taiwanese authorities described the recognition as a notable achievement, and a vindication of the strategy implemented after 2000 through the NGO Forum, its significance should not be exaggerated.

NGOs recognized by the UNDPI have only a relatively modest level of interaction with the UN. They are not as widely recognized as NGOs accredited with the ECOSOC or other UN agencies. In a way, it is a painful reminder of the discrimination of the UN system against Taiwanese organizations. Because of its global presence and remarkable achievements, in particular in the social, medical and humanitarian fields, Tzu Chi would be an obvious candidate for official recognition by the ECOSOC, WHO and other UN agencies, if it were not originally a Taiwanese organization. In contrast, the Buddha's Light International Association

> was established in 1991 in Taiwan and later set up headquarters in Los Angeles. It is another religious organization important for its volunteers. The organization has a strong system in place for international exchange and it managed to expand in five continents, in over 60 different countries and with 121 volunteer teams. This is one of the few NGOs in Taiwan that developed within the local community but then became global. In 2003, the Association became a Special Advisor in the United Nations Economic and Social Council (ECOSOC) and it strives to achieve the United Nations Millennium Development Goals.
>
> (NGO Affairs Committee, 2006: 90)

The fact that Tzu Chi has not yet obtained such recognition and status from the United Nations Economic and Social Council (ECOSOC) highlights the limitation of the government's strategy of expanding Taiwan's international space through participation in international NGOs, as the passport to UN accreditation for worthy Taiwanese NGOs seems to be relocation to another country. Ironically, China itself acknowledges the value of Tzu Chi's contribution to disaster relief and humanitarian aid, as Tzu Chi was reportedly the first foundation allowed to register as a 'non-resident' foundation on the mainland (*China Post*, 28 February 2008).

Concluding comments

The norms that guide Taiwan's aid programmes in general are consistent with global norms. Taiwan behaves like a state and pursues goals in line with its specific situation. It is difficult for Taiwan to disclose country-specific aid outputs because of its situation. Insofar as the governance norms, actors, processes and outcomes differ from those of other donors, they mostly reflect Taiwan's specific situation and precarious status. In terms of processes, Taiwan stands out for the use of informal networks and connections.

Taiwan's response to medical and humanitarian challenges is limited, scattered and hampered by Taiwan's low recognition. Overall these contributions lack visibility. Globally, ODA commitments are increasing rapidly, while Taiwan's contribution remains flat. Taiwan's medical and humanitarian aid alone is not important and visible enough to trigger a wave of support among developing countries for its WHO bid.

In contrast with its contribution to multilateral development banks or its technical assistance to agriculture, Taiwan's medical and humanitarian aid does not appear to be organized strategically. Its impact could be improved, it is suggested here, through a strengthened institutional framework, increased resources and better focused programmes. Taiwan could have done more in the past and strategically planned its aid allocations. In recent years the Taiwanese authorities have been slow to respond to new developments and the rapidly evolving environments of both medical aid and disaster response. Besides, subordinating the delivery of humanitarian aid to diplomatic recognition harms both people in need of assistance and Taiwan's efforts to become an observer at the WHO.

8 Conclusion

A revisiting

Research questions and hypotheses revisited

Returning to the questions and hypotheses set out in Chapter 1, it is clear that Taiwan is actively involved in global systems in response to health developments and to natural or man-made disasters, using key governance elements identified in Chapter 2. It is involved strategically in ways that seek to advance its international standing and status. In the process, it invokes various global norms, and its aid programmes involve governance actors and organizations from the state, market and civil society alike.

The hypothesis that Taiwan uses all of the governance elements at its disposal to facilitate its integration in the global system is only verified in part. More accurately, Taiwan uses all of the elements at its disposal, but does not necessarily use them fully. Taiwan's actors involved in medical and humanitarian assistance have historically been linked through several types of arrangements, but the DPP paradoxically appeared to be less effective in mobilizing non-state actors than the KMT. In addition, Taiwanese authorities do not appear to make full use of available policy instruments, nor of the international linkages that a rapidly evolving aid system offers. Aid outputs lack focus and are hampered by Taiwan's use of sticks to punish allies that defect, such as the cancellation of medical cooperation programmes with Chad and Malawi. Aid outcomes lack visibility and it is not possible to ascertain clear improvements for the intended beneficiaries.

Does Taiwan use the global governance systems that seek to respond to diseases and disasters to advance strategically its particular interests? The hypothesis that Taiwan uses this global system to enhance its status in the global arena is confirmed, as its primary objective is international recognition. The main reason it gives for its official medical and humanitarian aid programme is to gain observer status at the World Health Organization. Taiwan points to its contribution as one of the key arguments in support of its WHO bid but aid outputs and outcomes remain unconvincing. In addition, the cancellation of medical missions for diplomatic reasons weakens this key argument.

Taiwan is an irregular state and the hypothesis that, as such, it uses elements of governance that seek to respond to diseases and disasters in ways that are different from those of other states is confirmed in part. Taiwan uses some governance elements in ways other states do. In particular, all states use governance norms selectively. In contrast, the nature of Taiwan's official or quasi-official aid actors is difficult to ascertain and Taiwanese non-state actors operate with additional constraints due to international isolation. Besides, Taiwan does not have access to all the policy instruments other states use, in particular physical instruments. Its irregular situation also leads to selective disclosure of aid activities, although China's level of disclosure is, for other reasons, even more limited. Very importantly, a key outcome which Taiwan seeks is global recognition as a state, an issue which regular states do not have to address.

Case analyses revisited

Taiwan's quest for global recognition: the WHO observership bid

In its struggle to achieve global recognition in general and observership at the WHO in particular, Taiwan refers to three sets of governance norms: political, scientific and humanitarian. Political norms include sovereignty, human rights and universality. Taiwan claims it is sovereign and has exercised control over a well-defined territory and population for more than half a century. Taiwan specifically says it does not invoke the sovereignty principle in its bid to become an observer at the World Health Assembly but did so when it applied for membership in 2007 and 2008. This lack of consistency undermines Taiwan's case.

In support of its campaign Taiwan refers to the principle of universality, but scores low on this count if one keeps in mind the intransigent attitude of the Republic of China against the participation of Communist countries in the WHO in the 1950s and 1960s. In addition, records show that in the 1950s and 1960s the Republic of China was far from being the active participant in the WHO it now claims to have been.

Taiwan strongly emphasizes human rights as a norm and specifically argues that 'health for all' means that Taiwanese people cannot be excluded from the WHO. Besides, Taiwan stresses that its WHO bid has a dual humanitarian dimension. Exclusion from the WHO increases suffering for Taiwanese and people elsewhere as Taiwan cannot provide all the aid it wants to offer.

While Taiwan argues that if it became an observer at the WHO, people in Taiwan and elsewhere would be better off, the conclusion reached here is that it would hardly make any difference. Health indicators for Taiwan are already among the highest in the world. While Taiwan emphasizes that the aid it provides to developing countries, in particular in the medical and humanitarian fields, should be acknowledged, non-participation in the WHO does not prevent Taiwan from providing medical assistance to developing countries. Taiwan is on considerably firmer ground when it condemns the exclusion of Taiwanese journalists from the World Health Assembly. Nonetheless, there are pressing public health arguments to include Taiwan in substantive cooperation on epidemiological surveillance, in particular through the GOARN.

The three cases Taiwan cites most often as examples of its suffering due to exclusion from the WHO are unconvincing. There is no evidence that the WHO could have been more helpful if Taiwan had been an observer during the enterovirus outbreak. The WHO certainly would not have been able to do more in the aftermath of the Chi-Chi earthquake in 1999 as natural disasters are outside its competence. Taiwan failed to acknowledge the WHO's support during the SARS episode. The use of such arguments therefore highlights Taiwan's desperation more than its supposed virtue. Nonetheless, emphasizing health as a fundamental right appears to serve Taiwan's interests well. In particular, Taiwan's bid to become an observer at the WHO received support from the US, Japan, the European Parliament and the largest international medical associations.

The requirements of event-based coalitions, such as Taiwan's WHO campaign and its once-a-year high point, may be looser than those of a partnership focusing on service delivery. While Taiwanese medical activists and the government are clearly in touch, there is no apparent link between international medical associations and Taiwan's diplomatic allies, even though they support the same cause.

The Taiwanese authorities have not maximized the use of the policy instruments at their disposal in this regard. Taiwan was not interested in gaining recognition, and eventually access to the WHO, through low-key contributions or mechanisms like TDR or the Global Fund. This suggests that the primary, unstated objectives of the campaign contradict the official ones – except in 2007 and 2008 when Taiwan applied for membership. Beyond participating in the WHO as an observer, the point may be to satisfy a domestic audience and keep the Taiwan issue alive in international fora. Nonetheless, Taiwan could eventually, as a by-product of the campaign, reach its stated objective of becoming an observer under certain circumstances, such as an overwhelming public health emergency, should China fail to respond adequately. Statutorily, a simple majority of members or an invitation from the Director-General is required. Needless to say, such an invitation is unlikely to be extended against China's will during Margaret Chan's mandate, but it would be very difficult for any Director-General to make such a controversial decision anyway. Becoming an observer could be a first step towards WHO membership and onward to the UN.

China has a wide range of options and instruments at its disposal to counter Taiwan's bid. China is a nuclear power, a permanent member of the UN Security Council and an economic superpower. China has eroded Taiwan's diplomatic alliances and successfully isolated Taiwan in the international arena. But China does not have the power to prevent any country from raising the Taiwan issue at the Health Assembly. No prediction is offered here with regard to the outcome, but relevant governance processes are likely to be affected as long as the issue of Taiwan's participation in the global health governance system is not solved to the satisfaction of both sides of the Strait. In 2004 the Taiwan issue derailed the World Health Assembly. Some participants blamed Taiwan and its allies, others China and its allies. Accepting Taiwan's participation in WHO technical meetings was a way for China to deal with the criticism. It was also an acknowledgement that ignoring the human rights norm Taiwan invoked did not bolster its own position. The MoU China signed with the WHO opened a window to Taiwan's participation in WHO technical meetings and the possibility for the WHO to send experts to Taiwan in case of a public health emergency. Particular disputes can have lasting consequences for much wider governance processes. The WHO's policy for civil society organizations was affected by the China/Taiwan divide. The entire process of updating the policy stalled and the reworking of the policy was shelved.

The competition for influence over norm-setting takes the form of a selective invocation. As an example, the US recognizes China's sovereignty but does not support the view that it is good enough an excuse to disregard the human rights of Taiwanese people. Major powers invoke or fail to defend a specific norm or norms in a given 'battle' or episode. When Taiwan's major allies remain silent at the World Health Assembly, China prevails. When the US and Japan assert the inalienable right of Taiwanese people to health, Taiwan advances. While major powers can choose which norm to invoke at a given time, small countries dependent on Taiwan's aid or those fearful of China's clout have less room to manoeuvre.

Conversely, Taiwan receives only few of the benefits that regular states derive from complying with global norms. Taiwan cannot blackmail the WHO and threaten to behave dangerously or irresponsibly if it is not accepted as an observer.

Taiwan's medical and humanitarian assistance

Although they insist health is a right, Taiwanese officials do not focus clearly on the many people worldwide who lack access to effective healthcare. While they refer to the Millennium Declaration, the findings of the Commission on Macroeconomics and Health and other global aid norms, aid officials fail to articulate these norms in their medical and humanitarian assistance.

While referring to effectiveness and transparency, Taiwan discloses little about its aid programmes. Officials say they are anxious to avoid competition from the PRC and competitive bidding among their own allies. In spite of the DPP's insistence, ahead of the 2000 presidential election, on the need for an informed public debate about aid practices, programmes and disbursements, the level of transparency remained low, even in the case of medical and humanitarian aid. Old habits die hard.

Taiwanese humanitarian NGOs are restricted by the PRC in overseas operations and heavily constrained the Taiwanese government. The Tzu Chi Foundation can, more easily than smaller humanitarian organizations, choose when to work independently and when to collaborate with the government. Taiwanese humanitarian organizations apparently receive very little support from state organizations and are not really involved as meaningful partners.

This points to unexpected conclusions with regard to the use of policy instruments. The range of policy instruments at the disposal of Taiwan's government is rather limited, in particular physical instruments. Taiwan cannot send its Navy or its Air Force to rescue victims of disasters in the region. Taiwan's government cannot even secure visas for Taiwanese aid workers heading to countries which have no diplomatic links, whether official or unofficial, with Taiwan. As Taiwan has no existence in any of the UN agencies specialized in medical or humanitarian affairs, it is surprising that Taiwan is far from making full use of the policy instruments at its disposal, in particular material instruments.

Taiwan claims it is not as wealthy as other OECD donors and therefore has a lower ratio of ODA to GDP. The aid figures Taiwan provides raise several issues. Transparency is low and aggregate figures are questionable. It is not clear on what basis aid-in-kind is valued, be it medical supplies or food aid. Taiwan's economic aid is overwhelmingly provided in the forms of loans and it is unclear whether the loans Taiwan provides qualify as ODA.

Taiwan's government funding of NGOs for humanitarian operations overseas lacks transparency. Independent audits of joint operations, as in the cases of Afghanistan, Iraq and the Indian Ocean tsunami would help clarify the respective contributions of the state and non-state actors and organizations involved. In such cases, there is no excuse such as 'avoiding a bidding war with allies' or 'avoiding giving sensitive information to the enemy (i.e. the Peoples' Republic)' that makes sense.

While Taiwan's official contributions to multilateral development banks and agricultural development are noted, the instruments it uses to respond to disasters and public health crises appear to be ineffective. Part of the problem may be the poor devising and packaging of these instruments. Also, NGOs are reluctant to accept government funding, because they are wary of what they might be asked in return. There is hardly any transparency and predictability in the process.

This suggests that the low level of intake of material instruments also derives from the poor quality of linking arrangements, both among government agencies and between government agencies and NGOs. There is no clear process that links the political experience of the Ministry of Foreign Affairs, the project management experience of the ICDF and the medical expertise of the Department of Health, even though the establishment of TaiwanIHA in 2006 may lead to improvements.

The practical way Taiwan chose when it decided to channel its donation to the polio campaign through Rotary International helped it gain recognition and visibility. However, the Taiwanese government failed to replicate this success in the cases of the Global Fund contribution and the Chad/UNAIDS project. On the one hand the global aid scene has evolved and on the other hand Taiwanese authorities have failed to involve civil society. Or to put it in another way, whereas the linking arrangements of the KMT in the 1990s were effective in bringing together state and non-state actors to make the polio campaign a success, these arrangements were not replaced by equally effective ones. Taiwan was slow to adjust to changes in the governance systems handling responses to disasters and the global disease burden.

Taiwan's low level of material aid may appear to confirm that in a democracy, the tendency will be first to use the least intrusive policy instruments (i.e. symbolic instruments). But symbolic instruments alone hardly make any difference in the lives of people affected by illness and disasters. Overemphasis on symbolic instruments, at the expense of material ones, can eventually be counterproductive.

Does Taiwan's aid in the medical and humanitarian fields make a difference? Does it result in improved outcomes for the intended beneficiaries? The impact of Taiwan's medical and humanitarian assistance on beneficiaries is difficult to measure because of limited disclosure and a lack of focus, but can be assessed against the objective of raising Taiwan's profile in the international arena and entering the WHO. While the main stated objective of Taiwan's official humanitarian and medical aid programmes is to join the WHO, the number of Taiwan's medical missions in Africa was cut in half following the defection of Chad in 2006 and Malawi in 2008. Taiwan's international medical assistance overall fails to bring long-term benefits for patients and in diplomatic terms.

While Taiwan uses all the governance elements at its disposal to facilitate its global integration, it does so in varying measures. Taiwan selectively refers to governance norms relevant to medical and humanitarian aid and involves diverse categories of actors. But the Taiwanese authorities have limited interactions with non-governmental organizations and do not maximize the use of the policy instruments at their disposal.

Three paradoxes

The findings of the two case studies point to three paradoxes. The first paradox is that the single-minded, overriding objective of Taiwan's aid policy is to enter the WHO, which has had a decreasing role in meeting the objective of 'health for all'. On the one hand, the WHO campaign was started several years after Taiwan's bid to be readmitted in the United Nations and predicated on a different, though not unrelated argument: Taiwan focuses on the WHO's stated mission to defend the human rights of all people, including Taiwanese, and thus fulfil its mandate to achieve health for all in the twenty-first century. But over time the WHO lost part of its clout to other agencies including the World Bank, UNAIDS and the Global Fund.

The second paradox is that Taiwan seeks to co-opt NGOs and take credit for their achievements to the point of constraining their actions or making them look suspicious to outsiders, yet generally fails to consult and involve them in substantive ways. Officials thus miss opportunities to strengthen the impact and visibility of their own programmes. Taiwan tries to co-opt both businesses and NGOs in its efforts to achieve greater recognition. Humanitarian organizations are particularly attractive targets because of their positive image and outreach. But the Taiwanese government is so eager to capitalize on the positive image and achievements of humanitarian organizations for short-term gains that it takes the risk of jeopardizing diplomatic gains and greater global recognition in the longer term. It is surprising that the Taiwanese government has not sought to involve these organizations in more meaningful ways.

The third paradox is that even though Taiwan's government talks of a global, post-modern world where borders will supposedly become less and less relevant, it was slow to respond to the rapid evolutions of the governance systems that seek to tackle disasters and diseases. In particular, Taiwan aid officials long failed to understand, or chose to ignore, the many ways in which the WHO gathers and disseminates knowledge and expertise and generally interacts with the world. Increased disclosure, improved aid practices, better focused medical aid programmes, enhanced participation in donors' forums and a more skilful insertion in global aid dynamics would help Taiwan get more bang for its bucks. But it is also clear that Taiwan's government will have to scale up the resources it allocates to medical aid programmes if it wants to raise visibility and recognition to the levels it claims to have reached.

Taiwan and irregular states revisited

Is Taiwan's quest for status and recognition an elusive one? Taiwan positions itself as a state, or at least as an aspiring state, and seeks increased recognition as such. In this endeavour, Taiwan is in the company of other states. France's '*besoin de rayonnement*' was mentioned. Countries seeking a permanent seat on the UN Security Council, such as Japan and India, have also used aid to this effect (*Far Eastern Economic Review*, 2005). Even countries seeking a non-permanent, two-year stint on the UN Security Council have been shown, as in the case of the Netherlands, to spend political capital and flex financial aid muscle to this effect (Malone, 2000). Enhancing status is regarded by many states as national interest, even among permanent members of the Security Council. In seeking to improve its status through official aid programmes, Taiwan behaves like a state. Taiwan's low status is not the issue: Taiwan's assistance, in particular in the medical and humanitarian fields, is simply predicated on its right to exist in the global arena.

Taiwan portrays itself as both a helpless victim and a frustrated rescuer. Taiwan's atypical situation throws light on humanitarianism as a unique governance complex. While states often use, where applicable, one posture or the other (victim or rescuer), Taiwan consistently uses both at all times. It could be interesting to explore similarities and differences with discourses of other irregular states. States were found to participate, in response to crises, in a 'sacrificial international order' through intervention, involvement or abstention, and in particular the provision or denial of assistance (Bradol, 2004). While Taiwan's status certainly prohibits it from getting involved in humanitarian interventions, Taiwan was shown to participate in this sacrificial order through 'humanitarian withdrawal'.

Taiwan refers to sovereignty in ways which are necessarily different from those of regular states. The sovereignty claims of irregular/unrecognized states necessarily have a different subtext and are often regarded with suspicion by recognized states. Human rights have been used selectively by Taiwan and primarily portrayed as the human rights of Taiwanese people. The human rights of people elsewhere, in particular the citizens of Taiwan's allies and aid recipients, do not appear to have been taken into consideration seriously except when they serve Taiwan's drive for global recognition. One clear example is when Taiwan says it could provide more medical or humanitarian aid to developing countries if it were given observer status at the WHO. Taiwan's reference to human rights is afflicted with myopia. Unlike many countries, including current and former diplomatic allies, Taiwan enjoys prosperity and peace, thanks to the security guarantees of the US. But it can be argued that many states refer to the same principles in ways which are no less biased.

The China–Taiwan issue can be recast in part as a conflict between two norms: sovereignty and human rights. Even though all major powers dispute neither China's sovereignty nor its claim over Taiwan, many countries are critical of China's human rights record. Non-respect of human rights is a liability for China. Taiwan's case for WHO observership thrives on this weakness, as Taiwan decisively casts health as an inalienable human right. But Taiwan undermines its own case when it overlooks the consequences of an abrupt 'humanitarian withdrawal' as in Malawi.

Because of its unclear status, Taiwan has been very creative when it comes to describing itself. Sovereignty is sometimes emphasized as in the 'state-to-state relations' formula with regard to the PRC or when it is argued that there is no need to declare independence as Taiwan is already de facto independent. Taiwan behaves like a state in many respects but sometimes in ways other states don't. Taiwan has not ruled out unconventional avenues to promote its claims. In particular, Taiwanese authorities have explored alternative ways and forums along the line of non-governmental organizations, as in the examples of the Unrepresented Nations and Peoples' Organizations (UNPO) and the Democratic Pacific Union (DPU). In other cases, though, Taiwan describes itself neither as a state nor as a non-state organization, but shelves sovereignty claims to facilitate membership in international organizations as a functional entity. This was in particular the case with APEC, which Taiwan joined as an 'economy', and the WTO, where it was accepted as a 'customs territory'. To build up on the theme Taiwan now proposes to become an observer at the WHO as a 'health entity', a designation unknown to WHO statutes. In addition, Taiwan joined various maritime organizations and conventions as a 'fishing entity'. This is probably, though surely not intentionally, the best metaphor for an entity that keeps 'fishing' for a status and on the way resists attempts to be categorized by political scientists. It is interesting that Taiwan describes itself in different ways – state, NGO, functional entity – depending on the objectives it pursues.

Taiwan's aid actors' resemblance with counterparts in other countries is somewhat misleading. TaiwanICDF does not quite look like an official aid agency, but more like a development bank with a large corporate philanthropy programme. Businesses are involved in aid programmes and activities in roles that exceed what is normally expected from 'good corporate citizens'. NGOs are co-opted, as the government seeks in particular to raise the island's global profile through the increased interaction of NGOs with the UN and their affiliation with UN-accredited INGOs. In addition, Taiwan sometimes creates non-governmental organizations and entrusts them with varying levels of state authority or quasi-statutory tasks, as in the case of the Taiwan–Tibet Foundation and the Taiwan–Mongolia Association. Taiwan appears to do this more systematically than regular states. Its status has an impact on the characteristics of the organizations it interacts with and seems conducive to the breeding of hybrid forms.

Not all Taiwanese non-state actors side with the government. Most Taiwanese businessmen support China's efforts to block the island's moves towards independence. Taiwanese humanitarian NGOs struggle hard to defend their independence, while authorities make extensive use of their achievements.

Taiwan's irregular status, though, makes it even more imperative for the island to focus its aid on well-defined priorities and programmes with measurable outcomes if it wants to increase recognition and raise its status globally. In particular, Taiwan's medical and humanitarian aid alone is not important and visible enough to trigger a wave of support among developing countries for its WHO bid. In addition, unlike in the case of economic aid or agricultural aid, Taiwan's medical and humanitarian aid does not appear to be organized strategically. Its impact could be improved through a strengthened institutional framework, increased resources and better-focused programmes.

Lack of recognition certainly restricts Taiwan's capacity to provide aid, as it remains a non-entity for the main UN agencies involved in the response to disease and disaster. But Taiwan could be more proactive in organizations that are not part of the UN system, such as the Global Fund, where Taiwan already has donor and country adviser status, or the Development Aid Committee of the OECD.

Taiwan's ability to use physical instruments is constrained by its status, while China uses physical and material instruments to lure Taiwan's official diplomatic allies. These include offering peacekeeping forces, vetoing UN assistance to Taiwan's diplomatic allies, outbidding Taiwan in terms of aid pledges or trying to prevent Taiwan's diplomatic allies from sitting on the UN Security Council. But these actions only address part of the problem, as non-official allies of Taiwan, such as Japan or the United States, could keep the observership bid going even if Taiwan lost all its official allies. The US can speak in favour of Taiwan at the World Health Assembly without fearing retaliation from China. There is no foolproof method for China to completely offset the influence of human rights norms in global governance in general and the negative impact of its own record in this regard.

Another important feature of Taiwan's interaction with the world as an irregular state is its reliance on personal contacts and connections. The extent of Taiwan's private or unofficial diplomacy has been studied and established, in particular in Southeast Asia. This study shows that Tzu Chi in particular systematically tries to involve Taiwanese businessmen established overseas in its activities. The personal connection between the Taiwanese Minister of Health and his US counterpart appears to have led to strengthened support for Taiwan's

WHO bid and Taiwan's donation to the Global Fund. Without the personal connection between the Head of Tzu Chi's emergency operations and the General Manager of CARE-France, support from the Ministry of Foreign Affairs for the AIDS project in Chad would have been unlikely. The extent and impact of these personal contacts and connections are significant and point to an important issue: how far do they determine Taiwan's policy in the areas studied here? How far are an irregular state's choices constrained by its isolation?

The new 'people's diplomacy' emphasized by the Chen Shui-bian administration was supposed to help Taiwanese NGOs raise their profile with the UN. While the number of Taiwanese NGOs affiliated with UN-accredited INGOs has grown steadily, Tzu Chi's recognition by the 'low-level' United Nation's Department of Public Information (DPI) as an NGO with a significant information programme is not really the success story Taiwanese officials have tried to depict. It can be argued that the episode highlights the discrimination of the UN system against Taiwanese organizations. Because of its global presence and track record, Tzu Chi would obviously qualify for official accreditation with the ECOSOC, the WHO and other UN agencies, if it were not a Taiwan-based organization. In contrast, Buddha's Light International Association, which originated from Taiwan but relocated to Los Angeles in 1991, was accredited by ECOSOC in 2003. This certainly points to problems with the government's stated strategy of expanding Taiwan's global profile through the internationalization of local NGOs.

In both case studies, there is no evidence that the common good is maximized. Taiwan's aid programmes have a suboptimal impact in this regard both because the rest of the world ignores Taiwan and because Taiwan is not single-mindedly focused on maximizing what is generally perceived as the common good. Taiwan's main motive for its aid programmes is to enhance its international profile and global recognition. Taiwan's unusually generous aid package in the aftermath of the 2004 Indian Ocean tsunami suggests that an irregular state's choice of policy instruments, when addressing a global issue, may be informed not just by the democratic 'path of least resistance', but also by peer pressure (i.e. the behaviour of other states and global norms).

This research leads to more questions than answers on the Taiwan issue. What is Taiwan? As it behaves like a state, at least in the area studied here, should we suggest it is a state? Or a 'quasi-state'? Is it a 'like unit' in the neorealist sense? Is Taiwan more likely than its neighbours or other states elsewhere to disappear as a self-governing entity? Is the Peoples' Republic the main threat to Taiwan's existence as a self-governing entity? Or is it Taiwan's fractured polity?

It is difficult to think of any other state or aspiring state that presents similar characteristics. With the end of the apartheid and the Pinochet regime, both South Africa and Chile fully reintegrated the community of nation-states. Even Israel was never confronted with the same level of diplomatic isolation. The Taiwan case therefore seems to have either historical or limited relevance for other irregular states (i.e. states that enjoy a low level of international recognition). Taiwan's situation differs markedly from the situation of failed states such as

Afghanistan, the Democratic Republic of Congo, Myanmar, Liberia, Somalia and others. Palestine may be the closest case of an aspiring state, after Kosovo gained independence. But Palestine or Kosovo do not have the material resources at the disposal of Taiwan, and it remains to be seen whether Palestine would think of unconventional ways to reinforce statehood claims.

While other unrecognized states or states with low recognition may share Taiwan's conundrum and see human rights as the best way to strengthen their case for legitimacy, they do not necessarily enjoy Taiwan's level of control and effectiveness. This appears to validate the idea developed in Chapter 2 that a more suitable categorization of states and state sovereignty should include three dimensions:

- control (effective states/failed states);
- attitude towards human rights (legitimacy/illegitimacy);
- external sovereignty (recognition/isolation).

States could be mapped and graded along three main dimensions of statehood: states are more or less effective, more or less legitimate, more or less recognized.

Governance and governance theory revisited

Some final, overall ideas and questions are worth revisiting with regard to 'governance' and 'governance theory'. They suggest some possible lines of further theory development.

As participants in governance systems pursue their own interests and not just the common good, the architecture and characteristics of the system are affected in several ways. Compromises may be found, but power politics may also paralyse the system. Coalitions of actors of various types may form around issues on the basis of shared interests. Such coalitions may be fluid and the levels of commitment of the various participants may differ. In addition, and importantly, interests are often disguised as norms or ideas which have a broader appeal. Coalitions based on norms or ideas may be broader than those focused on narrowly defined interests.

The evolution of a global governance system over time depends on its ability to address the global issues it is meant to tackle. A governance system that delivers outputs and outcomes in line with the expectations of participants is likely to remain stable over time. Governance systems that seek to respond to diseases and disasters frequently do not operate in ways that satisfy key participants and stakeholders. Disappointing outcomes can result in significant levels of dissatisfaction, which in turn lead to the creation of new actors or the development of new processes. More research is needed on the extent to which global governance systems meet the expectations of participants and other stakeholders in various policy areas.

It is important to map the outcomes really targeted against the objectives and expectations of participants in various governance systems and arenas. In the global arena, governance is not just about maximizing the common good, whether one sees it in democratic or utilitarian terms. Governance also represents a system that entities or organizations can use to advance their own agenda, be it state interest, private profit or other. What improvement, if any, is targeted or achieved and for whom? Targeted outcomes are difficult to ascertain. They may be clearly stated in some cases and remain unstated in others. This in turn may affect the relevance of the analysis in terms of governance elements. One solution to this problem would be to start by ascertaining what the targeted outcome is in a given governance arrangement, and then move backwards. The mapping of outcomes and expectations, where feasible, would be key to assessing the relevance of governance processes and outputs. But participants in an arrangement may have in mind very diverse expectations.

Actors in a governance system often portray their interests as norms and invoke them selectively. There are several reasons why a selective invocation of norms may help actors enhance their position. Concealing targeted outcomes behind norms, values and principles may have advantages. Under the banner of ideas, it may be easier to involve people and organizations that would fail to spontaneously support one's interests. The selective invocation of norms may also push opponents to state on what basis they oppose suggested processes or targeted outcomes. Appealing to norms/values/ideas is more likely to broaden a coalition than appealing to one's sheer interests. Norm-broking then becomes an important aspect of tool selection.

In a conflict between two norms, principles or ideas, one should not overlook the distribution of physical and material capabilities among the actors behind the norms or the ideas. Governance actors are in part guided, and in part constrained, by existing governance norms. In this regard, powerful actors appear to have more latitude than others. Governance actors assign specific values (in the sense of valuations) to these norms. One measure of the power of ideas may be the weightings or at least the rankings that the various actors assign to particular ideas (i.e. first and foremost, the weightings or rankings that the most powerful actors assign to these ideas). Obviously, further research is needed on this aspect, but it is suggested here that the governance approach to the global arena appears to best integrate the views of both realists and constructivists in IR theory.

While states remain the central governance actors, non-state actors, be they business coalitions or civil society networks, are also important sources of norms. From the anti-slavery movement of the nineteenth century to recent campaigns including the international campaign to ban landmines or the campaign to promote access to life-saving drugs, non-state actors have challenged the sovereign rights of states to conduct 'business as usual'.

Governance actors influence and select processes. Powerful actors have more room to manoeuvre in this regard, but in some cases even weaker actors can influence processes. There is only limited evidence that norms influence the way linking arrangements are organized. Such arrangements are primarily based on convenience, acceptability, compromise and interest, even where actors agree on norms. The choice of linking arrangements results from the interaction of actors and norms, but parties to a linking arrangement do not have to agree on values and principles. Coalitions evolve and unravel over time in the global governance arena. Where few rules are written, the power of powerful actors is likely increased. Global or external non-state actors impact governance processes nearly everywhere, but even non-state actors in a national setting do not necessarily side with their own government. They are not just mechanical extensions of state actors.

As different types of actors have different strong points, including different types of actors in a coalition may enhance its effectiveness. States alone may not be able to convince that their main concern is the provision of global public goods. Businesses alone may not be able to convince that they care for more than shareholders' interests. Civil society organizations alone, whatever the strength of their transnational linkages, may not be able to muster the authority and material resources required to deliver the goods. It is also questionable whether all civil society organizations are single-mindedly focused on the provision of public goods.

This leads to the idea that actors of the same type are likely to cluster around distinctly identifiable norms or sets of norms. Integrating the lessons of various cases in global governance would help map these sets of norms more precisely. This does not mean, though, that a given norm, principle or set of norms is exclusive to one type of actors. Whereas it can be argued that sovereignty is the privilege of states, empirically all types of actors have been found to refer to human rights. All may also refer to a range of principles and norms including effectiveness, accountability, participation, justice and so on.

The credibility of these claims is open to debate. The legitimacy of each type of actor may be bound by a certain range of claims and predicated on an actor's focus on the intrinsic strengths of its category. An NGO's claim to be sovereign, a market organization's claim to be impartial or a state's claims to be an efficient entrepreneur may be received with scepticism.

There are infinite possibilities with regard to the use of policy instruments. The three-way categorization introduced in Chapter 2 makes sense in a crisis context, in particular the distinction between physical and material instruments. Many state and non-state actors respond to such crises with standard material instruments, such as blankets, food, medicines or plastic sheeting. But the instruments that make a real difference in emergency response are those not readily available on the market: an epidemiological surveillance network, a peacekeeping force, a cold chain for vaccines, trained sniffer dogs etc. No amount of material resources can be converted into such physical resources instantly, as is required in crisis situations.

Typologies are always helpful, but the key issue is the context. The toolbox should be assessed in the context of the workshop. One example is food aid. In most cases, it can be categorized as a material resource as food aid is monetized through food-for-work or food-for-development projects. But if food supplies dwindle drastically, which happens in particular in situations of conflict, the immediate survival of populations is at stake and food aid becomes a physical instrument, in the hands of relief workers as in the hands of warlords. Similarly, defining what constitutes valid official development assistance instruments and outputs has been an ongoing task for more than 40 years and there are still grey areas.

Symbolic instruments may be, as has been argued, the first choice of a democratic state in its panoply. Are they always appropriate? It probably depends on the objective being pursued. Symbolic instruments not backed up by a credible amount of physical or material instruments may have a limited impact. They may be cost-effective, but not necessarily effective. They may even be counter-productive. Again, understanding the context is key to devising an effective mix and packaging of instruments. China had the power to veto a UN mission to punish Macedonia, but was exposed as powerless as NATO intervened. China had the power to close its airspace to flights carrying relief, but undermined its argument that it cares for Taiwanese compatriots. Similarly Taiwan had the right to apply for WHO membership but undermined US support for its observer bid. And Taiwan had the capacity to withdraw its medical team from Malawi but levelled the moral high ground it was claiming to hold.

There is no reason to regard the use of instruments as the exclusive privilege of states. Non-state actors, whether for-profit or non-profit may too think in terms of physical, material and symbolic instruments to achieve their goals. This appears to be the case in particular in conflicts and other crisis situations where the state fails to deliver public goods such as security, and is an area for further research.

These ideas suggest wider questions with regard to the global arena. How far does the governance concept help make sense of the ways issues deemed of global interest, in particular crises, are addressed? Are the emerging patterns of global governance underpinned by recognized norms and the cooperation of most, if not all, organizations and other actors in helping to maximize the common good? Or are the patterns just a useful marker of the new constraints and opportunities states and other actors face in an increasingly complex world? Does governance just help map the relative power of all the actors involved? Or can it provide insights into innovative and potentially more effective ways to address global issues? These are questions that go beyond the focus of this study. It is hoped that they will help stimulate further research on the scope and potential of the governance approach in the global arena.

References

abcNews (30 September 2005) 'Expert predicts "perfect setup" for avian flu pandemic'. Online, available at: http://abcnews.go.com/GMA/Flu/story?id=1172638&page=1 (accessed 23 August 2008).

Agamben, Giorgio (1999) *Remnants of Auschwitz: the Witness and the Archive*, trans. Daniel Heller-Roazen. New York: Zone Books.

Agence France-Presse (12 November 2001) 'Taiwan–Chad–AIDS: Taiwan finances Chad's anti-AIDS project'.

Alger, Chadwick (2002) 'The emerging roles of NGOs in the UN system: from Article 71 to a people's millennium assembly'. *Global Governance* 8: 93–117.

Asia Pulse (3 January 2005) 'Taiwan offers US$50 MLN in relief aid to tsunami-hit countries'. Online, available at: http://asia.news.yahoo.com/050103/4/1u218.html (accessed 7 March 2005).

Australia–China Chamber of Commerce and Industry of New South Wales (2001) 'Ninth APEC Economic Leaders Meeting in Shanghai: what does it tell us about China?' Online, available at: www.accci.com.au/apec.htm (accessed 25 July 2006).

Badie, Bertrand (2002) 'Sovereignty and intervention in the post-September 11 world', Conference held on 3 October 2002 at the Convocation Room, Main Building, Main Campus, The University of Hong Kong.

Balaam, David N. and Veseth, Michael (1996; 2nd edn 2001) *Introduction to International Political Economy*. Upper Saddle River: Prentice Hall.

Batliwala, Srilatha (2002) 'Grassroots movements as transnational actors: implications for global civil society'. *Voluntas* 13: 393–409.

Beier, J. Marshall (2002) 'Siting indiscriminacy: India and the global movement to ban landmines'. *Global Governance* 8: 305–21.

Bellion-Jourdan, Jérôme (1997) 'L'humanitaire et l'islamisme soudanais' [Humanitarian aid and Sudanese Islamism]. *Politique africaine* 66: 61–73.

Bettati, Mario and Kouchner, Bernard (1987) *Le droit d'ingérence: peut-on les laisser mourir?* [The right to intervene: can we let them die?]. Paris: Denoël.

Bouchet-Saulnier, Françoise (2002) *The Practical Guide to Humanitarian Law*. First English Language edition. Edited and translated by Laura Brav. Lanham: Rowman & Littlefield.

Bradol, Jean- Hervé (2004) 'The sacrificial international order and humanitarian action'. In Weissman, Fabrice (ed.) *In the Shadow of 'Just Wars': Violence, Politics and Humanitarian Action. Médecins sans frontiers*. London: Hurst.

Brauman, Rony (1995) *L'action humanitaire* [Humanitarian Action]. Paris: Flammarion.

Brigham, John and Brown, Don W. (1980) 'Introduction'. In Brigham, John and Brown, Don W. (eds) *Policy Implementation: Penalties or Incentives?* Beverly Hills: Sage.

Brown, David L. and Moore, Mark H. (2001) 'Accountability, strategy, and international nongovernmental organizations'. *Nonprofit and Voluntary Sector Quarterly* 30: 569–87.

Brown, Kerry and Keast, Robyn (2003) 'Citizen-government engagement: community connection through networked arrangements'. *Asian Journal of Public Administration* 25: 107–31.

Brundtland, Gro Harlem (2001) 'Message from Director-General, 11 May 2001'. Geneva: World Health Organization.

Burci, Gian Luca and Vignes, Claude-Henri (2004) *World Health Organization*. The Hague: Kluwer Law International.

Burke, Edmund (1987) *Reflections on the Revolution in France*. New York: Prometheus Books.

Buse, Kent and Walt, Gill (2000) *The United Nations and Global Public-Private Health Partnerships: in Search of 'Good' Global Health Governance*. Paper presented at the workshop on Public–Private Partnerships in Public Health. Dedham, Massachusetts. 7–8 April 2000.

Cabestan, Jean-Pierre (2006) 'Marginalizing Taiwan weakens mainland security'. In Friedman, Edward (ed.) *China's Rise, Taiwan's Dilemmas and International Peace*. London: Routledge.

Cairo Declaration (1943) *Declaration of the Three Powers–Great Britain, the United States and China regarding Japan. Signed at Cairo, November 27, 1943*. Online, available at: www.ndl.go.jp/constitution/e/etc/c03.html (accessed 19 August 2006).

Caiveau, Hervé (2004) Interview with Hervé Caiveau, Paris, 13 June 2004.

Central Intelligence Agency (2006a) *World Factbook*. Online, available at: www.cia.gov/cia/publications/factbook/geos/tw.html (accessed 23 June 2006).

Central Intelligence Agency (2006b) *World Factbook*. Online, available at: www.cia.gov/cia/publications/factbook/geos/tp.html (accessed 13 July 2006).

Central News Agency (7 July 2002) 'ROC offers additional food aid to Malawi'. Online, available at: www.gio.gov.tw/taiwan-website/5-gp/africa2/abaf2a15.htm (accessed 26 August 2008).

Central News Agency (29 May 2005) 'China reveals contents of MOU on Taiwan–WHO technical exchanges'. Online, available at: www.globalsecurity.org/wmd/library/news/taiwan/2005/taiwan-050529-cna02.htm (accessed 26 August 2008).

Central News Agency (20 July 2005) 'Taiwan ranks 15th globally for world trade volume in 2004'. Online, available at: http://investintaiwan.nat.gov.tw/en/news/200507/2005072001.html (accessed 14 March 2006).

Chan, Gerald (1997a) 'Taiwan as an emerging foreign aid donor: developments, problems, and prospects'. *Pacific Affairs* 70: 37–56.

Chan, Gerald (1997b) '"Three Chinas" and international organizations after 1997'. *Journal of Contemporary China* 6: 435–48.

Chan, L. G., Parashar, U. D., Lye, M. S., Ong, F. G., Zaki, S. R., Alexander, J. P., Ho, K. K., Han, L. L., Pallansch, M. A., Suleiman, A. B., Jegathesan, M. and Anderson, L. J. (2000) 'Deaths of children during an outbreak of hand, foot and mouth disease in Sarawak, Malaysia: clinical and pathological characteristics of the disease'. *Clinical Infectious Diseases* 31: 678–83.

Chan, Steve (1998) *Keynote Address by C. Steve Chan M.D., Minister of Health, Taiwan, R.O.C. at the Reception of the Taiwan World Health Alliance*, 13 May 1998, Hotel Noga Hilton, Geneva. Online, available at: www.taipei.org/current/un/who-chan2.htm (accessed 23 July 2004).

Chang, Mau-kuei (2000) 'On the origins and transformation of Taiwanese national identity'. *China Perspectives* 28: 51–70.

Chang, Peter. (2004) Interview with Peter Chang, Advisor to the Ministry of Health, Taipei diplomatic mission, Geneva, 9 June 2004.

Chen, Homin and Liu, Meng-chun (1998) 'Noneconomic elements of Taiwan's foreign direct investment'. In Chen, Tain-jy (ed.) *Taiwanese Firms in Southeast Asia: Networking across Borders.* Cheltenham: Edward Elgar.

Chen, Jie (2002) *Foreign Policy of the New Taiwan: Pragmatic Diplomacy in Southeast Asia.* Cheltenham: Edward Elgar.

Chen, Solomon (2008) 'Medical mission in Malawi'. E-mail (28 August 2008).

Chen, Tain-jy (1998) 'Introduction'. In Chen, Tain-jy (ed.) *Taiwanese Firms in Southeast Asia: Networking across Borders.* Cheltenham: Edward Elgar.

Chen, Wen-deh (2006) 'Food aid'. E-mail (18 August 2006).

Cheng, Tung-jen (1995) 'The mainland China-Taiwan dyad as a research program'. In Cheng, Tun-jen and Huang, Chi (eds) *Inherited Rivalry: Conflict across the Taiwan Straits.* Boulder: Lynne Rienner.

China News Agency (23 September 1999) 'MAC dismisses Mainland Red Cross Society's claim'.

China News Agency (4 April 2005) 'Taiwan rejects WHO accession under "one China" framework'.

China Post (30 April 2004) 'DOH International Cooperation Unit expected to expand'.

China Post (8 November 2005) 'Officials decline to reveal aid to Senegal'. Online, available at: www.chinapost.com.tw/print/71559.htm (accessed 26 August 2008).

China Post (28 February 2008) 'Tzu Chi gets nod to set up charity in China'. Online, available at: www.chinapost.com.tw/taiwan/china-taiwan%20relations/2008/02/28/144823/Tzu-Chi.htm (accessed 2 September 2008).

Ching-long Lu, Michel (2004) Interview with Michel Ching-long Lu, Ambassador, Spokesman of the Ministry of Foreign Affairs, Taipei, 21 September 2004.

Chirac, Pierre and Torreele, Els (2006) 'Global framework on essential health R&D'. *The Lancet* 367: 1560–1.

Chiu, Hungdah (1979) 'Taiwan in Sino-American relations'. In Chiu, Hungdah (ed.) *China and the Taiwan issue.* New York: Praeger.

Chiu, Hungdah (1998) 'Taiwan and the United Nations'. In Glassner, Martin I. (ed.) *The United Nations at Work.* Westport: Praeger.

Chou, David S. (1999) 'The Washington–Taipei–Beijing strategic triangle'. In Chao, Chien-min and Clark, Cal (eds) *The ROC on the Threshold of the 21st Century: a Paradigm Reexamined.* Baltimore: University of Maryland School of Law.

Chu, Jou-juo (2001) *Taiwan at the end of the 20th Century: the Gains and Losses.* Taipei: Tonsan Publications.

Chu, Shulong and Guo, Yuli (2008) 'Change: Mainland's Taiwan policy'. *China Security* 4: 130–6.

Clough, Ralph N. (1999) *Cooperation or Conflict in the Taiwan Strait?* Lanham: Rowman & Littlefield.

CNN.com (8 June 1998) 'Child-killing virus baffles Taiwan'. Online, available at: www.cnn.com/WORLD/asiapcf/9806/08/taiwan.deadly.virus/ (accessed 27 July 2004).

Cohen, Robin and Rai, Shirin M. (2000) 'Towards a cosmopolitan politics'. In Cohen, Robin and Rai, Shirin M. (eds) *Global Social Movements.* London: Athlone Press.

Colonomos, Ariel (2001) 'Non-state actors as moral entrepreneurs: a transnational perspective on ethics networks'. In Josselin, Daphné and Wallace, William (eds) *Non-state Actors in World Politics*. New York: Palgrave.

Council of Agriculture (2004) 'Holistic development of agriculture, enhancing farmers' and fishermen's welfare'. In *Annual Report 2004*. Online, available at: http://eng.coa.gov.tw/./content.php?catid=10201&hot_new=10168 (accessed 12 August 2006).

Cuny, Frederick C. (1993) 'Humanitarian assistance in the Post-Cold War era'. In Weiss, Thomas and Minear, Larry (eds) *Humanitarianism across Borders: Sustaining Civilians in Times of War*. Boulder: Lynne Rienner.

Deng, Francis M. (1993) *Protecting the Dispossessed: a Challenge for the International Community*. Washington, DC: Brookings Institution.

Deng, Ping (2000) 'Taiwan's restriction of investment in China in the 1990s: a relative gains approach'. *Asian Survey* 40: 958–80.

Department of Humanitarian Affairs (1997) DHA-87: 1:14-Oct-97. Liberia Humanitarian Situation Report No. 87. 1–14 October 1997.

DeWaal, Alex (1997) *Famine Crimes: Politics and the Disaster Relief Industry*. African Issues. Oxford: James Currey.

Dierks, Leif (2004) Interview with Leif Dierks, IFRC, Taipei, 22 September 2004.

Donini, Antonio (1995) 'The bureaucracy and the free spirits: stagnation and innovation in the relationship between the UN and NGOs'. *Third World Quarterly* 16: 421–39.

Drahos, Peter and Braithwaite, John (2001) 'The globalisation of regulation'. *Journal of Political Philosophy* 9: 103–28.

Duffield, Mark (1997) 'NGO relief in war zones: towards an analysis of the new aid paradigm'. *Third World Quarterly* 18: 527–42.

Duffield, Mark (2001) *Global Governance and the New Wars: the Merging of Development and Security*. London: Zed Books.

Easton, David (1953) *The Political System: An Inquiry into the State of Political Science*. New York: Alfred A. Knopf.

Easton, David (1965) *A Systems Analysis of Political Life*. NewYork: John Wiley & Sons.

Edwards, Michael and Hulme, David (eds) (1996) *Beyond the Magic Bullet: NGO Performance and Accountability in the Post Cold War World*. West Hartford: Kumarian.

Etzioni, Amitai (1975) *A Comparative Analysis of Complex Organisations*. New York: Free Press/Macmillan.

Evans, Peter B., Skocpol, Theda and Rueschemeyer, Dietrich (eds) (1985) *Bringing the State back in*. Cambridge: Cambridge University Press.

Fanchiang, Cecilia (11 April 2003) 'Taiwan a major contributor to world health'. Online, available at: http://taiwanjournal.nat.gov.tw/ct.asp?xItem=19956&CtNode=122 (accessed 25 August 2008).

Far Eastern Economic Review (2005) 'Tokyo's quixotic quest for acceptance'. May 2005. 168: 5–10.

Fell, Dafydd (2004) 'Measurement of party position and party competition in Taiwan'. *Issues and Studies* 40: 101–36.

Feng, Joyce Y. (1999) 'Taiwan'. In T. Silk (ed.) *Philanthropy and Law in Asia: a Comparative Study of the Nonprofit Legal Systems in Ten Asia Pacific Societies*. San Francisco: Jossey-Bass.

Fichte, Johann Gottlieb (1978) *Reden an die deutsche Nation* [Discourse to the German Nation]. Hamburg: Meiner.

Finkelstein, Neal D. (2000) 'Introduction: transparency in public policy'. In Finkelstein, Neal D. (ed.) *Transparency in Public Policy: Great Britain and the United States.* London: Macmillan.

Flanders, Laura (1999) 'Giving The Vatican The Boot'. Online, available at: www.seechange.org/media/ms%20magazine%2010%2099.htm (accessed 22 August 2008).

Florini, Ann (ed.) (2000) *The Third Force: the Rise of Transnational Civil Society.* Tokyo: Japan Center for International Exchange, and Washington, DC: Carnegie Endowment for International Peace.

Formosan Association for Public Affairs (undated) *About FAPA.* Online, available at: www.fapa.org/main/about_fapa.htm (accessed 20 August 2006).

Forsythe, David P. and Rieffer-Flanagan, Barbara Ann J. (2007) *The International Committee of the Red Cross: a Neutral Humanitarian Actor.* London: Routledge.

Foucault, Michel (1997) *Il faut défendre la société* [Society must be Defended]: *Cours au Collège de France, 1975–1976.* Paris: Gallimard/Seuil.

Franceschet, Antonio (2002) 'Justice and international organization: two models of global governance'. *Global Governance* 8: 19–34.

Free China Journal (21 March 2003) 'Medical professional group targets WHO entry'. Online, available at: http://publish.gio.gov.tw/FCJ/past/03032121.html (accessed 26 August 2006).

Free China Journal (28 May 2004) 'Taiwan's 8th bid for WHA entry noticed'. Online, available at: http://publish.gio.gov.tw/FCJ/past/04052812.html (accessed 26 August 2006).

Free China Journal (6 August 2004) 'Taiwan contributes to MDG goals'. Online, available at: http://publish.gio.gov.tw/FCJ/past/04080662.html (accessed 30 June 2006).

Friends of Tibet (2003) 'Exile Government not involved with Taiwan group'. Online, available at: www.friendsoftibet.org/databank/tibetexile/tibete106.html (accessed 12 July 2006).

Fuchs, Doris A. (2004) 'The role of business in global governance'. In Schirm, Stefan (ed.) *New Rules for Global Markets: Public and Private Governance in the World Economy.* Basingstoke: Palgrave Macmillan.

Fukuyama, Francis (1992) *The End of History and the Last Man.* London: Penguin Books.

Gao, Pat (2004) 'Moving toward a better life'. Online, available at: www.gio.gov.tw/taiwan-website/5-gp/join_who/who35–09.htm (accessed 26 July 2004).

Garver, John W. (1997) *The Sino-American Alliance: Nationalist China and American Cold War Strategy in Asia.* Armonk: Sharpe.

Gazley, Beth and Brudney, Jeffrey L. (2007) 'The purposes (and perils) of government-nonprofit partnership'. *Nonprofit and Voluntary Sector Quarterly* 36: 389–415.

Geldenhuys, Deon (1990) *Isolated States: a Comparative Analysis.* Cambridge: Cambridge University Press.

Ghandour, Abdel-Rahman (2002) *Jihad humanitaire: enquête sur les ONG islamiques* [Humanitarian Jihad: a Survey of Islamic NGOs]. Paris: Flammarion.

Global Business Coalition (undated) Online, available at: www.businessfightsaids.org/site/pp.asp?c=nmK0LaP6E&b=202239 (accessed 20 February 2005).

Global Fund (2005) *The Global Fund's First Replenishment 2006–2007. Chair's Report.* Online, available at: www.theglobalfund.org/en/about/replenishment/london/default.asp (accessed 23 August 2006).

Global Fund (2006a) *Pledges.* Online, available at: www.theglobalfund.org/en/funds_raised/pledges/ (accessed 11 July 2006).

Global Fund (2006b) *Current Grants Commitments and Disbursements*. Online, available at: www.theglobalfund.org/en/funds_raised/commitments/ (accessed 24 April 2005).

Global Fund (2006c) *São Tomé and Príncipe and the Global Fund. Country Coordinating Mechanism*. Online, available at: www.theglobalfund.org/programs/CCMMembers.aspx?CountryId=STP&lang (accessed 15 July 2006).

Global Fund (undated) *Key Global Fund structures*. Online, available at: www.theglobalfund.org/en/about/structures/ (accessed 24 April 2005).

Global Polio Eradication Initiative (2006a) *Donor Contributions to the Global Polio Eradication Initiative 1985–2008*. Online, available at: www.polioeradication.org/poliodonors.asp (accessed 13 July 2006).

Global Polio Eradication Initiative (2006b) *Annual Expenditure 1988–2005. Financial Resource Requirement, Contributions, Funding Gap, 2006–2008*. Online, available at: www.polioeradication.org/fundingbackground.asp (accessed 13 July 2006).

Gong, Ting and Chen, Feng (1996) 'The rise of developmentalism across the Taiwan Strait'. In Yu, Bin and Chung, Tsungting (eds) *Dynamics and Dilemma: Mainland, Taiwan and Hong Kong in a Changing World*. New York: Nova Science Publishers.

Green, Daniel (2005) 'Liberal imperialism as global-governance perspective'. In Ba, Alice D. and Hoffmann, Matthew J. (eds) *Contending Perspectives on Global Governance: Coherence, Contestation and World Order*. London: Routledge.

Guilloux, Alain (2008) 'Regional governance and disaster response'. In *Governance and Regionalism in Asia*. London: RoutledgeCurzon.

Guilloux, Alain and Moon, Suerie (2000) *Hidden Price Tags. Disease-Specific Drug Donations: Costs and Alternatives*. Working group expert paper presented at the conference: 'The crisis of neglected diseases', Geneva, October 2000. Online, available at: www.neglecteddiseases.org/4–3.pdf (accessed 24 April 2005).

Hall, Rodney B. and Biersteker, Thomas J. (2002) 'The emergence of private authority in the international system'. In Hall, Rodney B and Biersteker, Thomas J. (eds) *The Emergence of Private Authority in Global Governance*. Cambridge: Cambridge University Press.

Hay, Colin and Lister, Michael (2006) 'Introduction: theories of the state'. In Hay, Colin, Lister, Michael and Marsh, David (eds) *The State: Theories and Issues*. Basingstoke: Palgrave Macmillan.

Hayek, Friedrich A. (1944) *The Road to Serfdom*. Chicago: University of Chicago Press.

Head, Brian and Ryan, Neal (2003) 'Working with non-government organisations: a sustainable development perspective'. *Asian Journal of Public Administration* 25: 31–56.

Health Taiwan (28 March 2003) 'MOFA calls coordination meeting for Iraqi refugee assistance'. Online, available at: http://healthtaiwan.doh.gov.tw/whowbs/article_post/post_userviewE_axtpg.jsp?ID_NO=224 (accessed 5 March 2005).

Hindmoor, Andrew (2006) 'Public choice'. In Hay, Colin, Lister, Michael and Marsh, David (eds) *The State: Theories and Issues*. Basingstoke: Palgrave Macmillan.

Ho, M., Chen, E. R., Hsu, K. H., Twu, S. J., Chen, K. T., Tsai, S. F., Wang, J. R. and Shih, S. R. (1999) 'An epidemic of enterovirus 71 infection in Taiwan'. *The New England Journal of Medicine* 341: 929–35.

Hobbes, Thomas (1996) *Leviathan*. Edited with an introduction by J. C. A. Gaskin. Oxford: Oxford University Press.

Hoffmann, Matthew J. and Ba, Alice D. (2005) 'Introduction: coherence and contestation'. In Ba, Alice D. and Hoffmann, Matthew J. (eds) *Contending Perspectives on Global Governance: Coherence, Contestation and World Order*. London: Routledge.

Hsiao, Hsin-huang Michael (1995) 'The growing Asia Pacific concern among Taiwan's NGOs'. In Yamamoto, Tadashi (ed.) *Emerging Civil Society in the Asia Pacific Community: Nongovernmental Underpinnings of the Emerging Asia Pacific Regional Community: a 25th Anniversary Project of JCIE.* Singapore: Institute of Southeast Asian Studies (ISEAS) and Asia Pacific Philanthropy Consortium (APPC).

Hsiao, Hsin-huang Michael (undated) *The Non-profit Sector in Taiwan: Current State, New Trend and Future Prospect.* Online, available at: www.tpic.org.tw/NPOInfo/index1–2.asp (accessed 2 August 2006).

Hsu, Hsiang-Ming (2004) Interview with Hsiang-Ming Hsu, Tzu Chi Foundation, Hualien, 24 September 2004.

Hsueh, Po-Ren and Yang, Pan-Chyr (2003) 'Severe Acute Respiratory Syndrome (SARS): an emerging infection of the 21st century'. *Journal of the Formosan Medical Association* 102: 825–39.

Huang, Julia C. (2002) 'What travels? Notes on a globalizing Buddhist movement from Taiwan'. *IWM Junior Visiting Fellows Conference*, Vol. XII/4. Online, available at: www.iwm.at/publ-jvc/jc-12–04.pdf (accessed 8 March 2005).

Huang, Sophia (2001) 'Taiwan's rice import market to open with WTO accession'. In *Rice Situation and Outlook Yearbook*/RCS-2001/Economic Research Service/USDA. Online, available at: http://72.14.203.104/search?q=cache:gF3wPuFaBtAJ:www.ers.usda.gov/Briefing/Rice/SpecialArticle/Taiwanrice.pdf+sophia+huang+taiwan+rice&hl=en&gl=hk&ct=clnk&cd=1 (accessed 15 July 2006).

Huang, Song-lih (2004) Interview with Song-lih Huang, Taiwan International Medical Alliance, Taipei, 22 September 2004.

Huang, Xiaoming (2001) 'Contested state and competitive state: managing the economy in a democratic Taiwan'. In Huang, Xiaoming (ed.) *The Political and Economic Transition in East Asia: Strong Market, Weakening State.* Richmond: Curzon.

Ignatieff, Michael (2002) 'Intervention and state failure'. *Dissent* 49: 115–23.

Inbar, Efraim (1985) *Outcast Countries in the World Community.* Monograph series in world affairs 21, 2. Denver: Graduate school of international affairs, University of Denver.

Initiative on Public–Private Partnerships for Health (IPPPH) (2004) 'Not-for-profit approach improves prospect of vaccines and drugs for the poor: US$2 billion investment yields significant progress, but more funders required'. Online, available at: www.ippph.org/index.cfm?page=/ippph/newsmedia/news&thechoice=show&id=521 (accessed 25 April 2005).

Jackson, Robert H. (1990) *Quasi-states: Sovereignty, International Relations and the Third World.* Cambridge: Cambridge University Press.

Jacoby, Neil H. (1966) *U.S. Aid to Taiwan: a Study of Foreign Aid, Self-help and Development.* New York: Praeger.

Jean, François (1996) 'Aide humanitaire et économie de guerre' [Humanitarian aid and war economics]. In Jean, François and Rufin, Jean-Christophe (eds) *Économie des guerres civiles* [The Economics of Civil Wars]. Paris: Hachette.

Kaul, Inge, Grunberg, Isabelle and Stern, Marc A. (1999) 'Defining global public goods'. In Kaul, Inge, Grunberg, Isabelle and Stern, Marc A. (eds) *Global Public Goods: International Cooperation in the 21st Century.* New York: Oxford University Press.

Keck, Margaret and Sikkink, Kathryn (1998) *Activists beyond Borders: Advocacy Networks in International Politics.* Ithaca: Cornell University Press.

Keohane, Robert O. and Nye, Joseph S. Jr (eds) (1971) *Transnational Relations and World Politics.* Cambridge: Harvard University Press.

Khagram, Sanjeev, Riker, James V. and Sikkink, Kathryn (eds) (2002) *Restructuring World Politics: Transnational Social Movements, Networks and Norms*. Minneapolis: University of Minnesota Press.

Kiwanis International (2007) *What is a Kiwanian?* Online, available at: www.kiwanis.org/WhoWeAre/WhatisaKiwanian/tabid/297/Default.aspx (accessed 19 August 2008).

Korea Times (4 April 2008) 'For global disease prevention'. Online, available at: www.koreatimes.co.kr/www/news/opinon/opi_view.asp?newsIdx=21964&categoryCode=197 (accessed 25 August 2008).

Ku, Samuel C. Y. (2002) 'The political economy of regime transformation: Taiwan and Southeast Asia'. *World Affairs* 165: 59–78.

Kuan, Eugene Hung-chang (2006) 'Domestic politics of foreign policy: explaining the formulation of Taiwan's "participate in the U.N." policy'. *Issues and Studies* 42: 137–62.

Kuo, Cheng-tian (1995) 'The political economy of Taiwan's investment in China'. In Cheng, Tun-jen and Huang, Chi (eds) *Inherited Rivalry: Conflict across the Taiwan Straits*. Boulder: Lynne Rienner.

Lam, Danny and Clark, Cal (1998) 'The cultural roots of "guerrilla capitalism" in Taiwan'. In Chan, Steve, Clark, Cal and Lam, Danny (eds) *Beyond the Developmental State: East Asia's Political Economies Reconsidered*. London: Macmillan.

Lebas, Pierre-Bernard (2004) Interview with Pierre-Bernard Lebas, UNHCR, Geneva, 9 June 2004.

Lee, Coral (2003) 'Taiwan bid for WHO participation again blocked by PRC'. Online, available at: www.sinorama.com.tw/en/show_issue.php3?id=200369206062e.txt&page=1 (accessed 23 July 2004).

Lee, Grace (2004) Interview with Grace Lee, Taiwan Root Medical Peace Corps, Taipei, 23 September 2004.

Lee, Stephen (2004) Interview with Stephen Lee, Deputy Director, Policy, Planning and Programming Department, TaiwanICDF, Taipei, 21 September 2004.

Leng, Tse-kang (1996) *The Taiwan-China Connection: Democracy and Development across the Taiwan Straits*. Boulder: Westview Press.

Lévêque, Philippe (2005) Interview with Philippe Lévêque, CARE-France, Paris, 10 June 2005.

Li, Christian (2004) Interview with Christian Li, Taiwan Red Cross, Taipei, 22 September 2004.

Liberty Times (27 October 2004) 'Medical mission a hit in Malawi; representatives attend WHO meeting'. Online, available at: http://english.www.gov.tw/TaiwanHeadlines/index.jsp?categid=11&recordid=78059 (accessed 15 July 2006).

Lien Fen Tseng, Wen Chun Chang, Maria Conceição Ferreira, Cheng Hua Wu, Herodes Sacramento Rampão and Jih Ching Lien (2008) 'Short report: rapid control of malaria by means of indoor residual spraying of alphacypermethrin in the Democratic Republic of São Tomé and Príncipe'. *American Journal of Tropical Medicine and Hygiene* 78: 248–50.

Lin, Chia-lung (2001) 'National identity and Taiwan security'. In Tan, Alexander C., Chan, Steve and Jillson, Calvin (eds) *Taiwan's National Security: Dilemmas and Opportunities*. Aldershot: Ashgate.

Lin, Teh-chang (2005) *An Assessment of Civil Society in Taiwan. Transforming State–Society Relations: the Challenge, Dilemma and Prospect of Civil Society in Taiwan*. Kaohsiung: Center for International NGO Studies, National Sun Yat-sen University.

Liu, Benjamin (2004). E-mail (donation to polio eradication campaign) (11 October 2004).

Liu, Benjamin (2004) Interview with Benjamin Liu, Department of International Organizations, Ministry of Foreign Affairs, Taipei, 22 September 2004.

Malone, David M. (2000) 'Eyes on the prize: the quest for nonpermanent seats on the UN Security Council'. *Global Governance* 6: 3–23.

Mandell, Myrna P. and Steelman, Toddi A. (2003) 'Understanding what can be accomplished through interorganizational innovations: the importance of typologies, context and management strategies'. *Public Management Review* 5: 197–224.

Masujima, Ken (2004) '"Good governance" and the Development Assistance Committee: ideas and organizational constraints'. In Bøås, Morten and McNeill, Desmond (eds) *Global Institutions and Development: Framing the World?* London: Routledge.

Mengin, Françoise (1999) 'State and identity'. In Tsang, Steve and Tien, Hung-mao (eds) *Democratization in Taiwan: Implications for China.* Hong Kong: Hong Kong University Press.

Mengin, Françoise (2007) 'A Tocquevillian process: Taiwan's democratization and its paradoxical foundations'. In Ash, Robert and Green, J. Megan (eds) *Taiwan in the 21st century: Aspects and Limitations of a Development Model.* London: Routledge.

Minear, Larry and Weiss, Thomas (1995) *Mercy under Fire: War and the Global Humanitarian Community.* Boulder: Westview Press.

Morris, Susannah (2000) 'Defining the non-profit sector: some lessons from history'. *Voluntas* 11: 25–43.

Mumford, Stephen D (1992) *The Vatican and World Population Policy: An Interview with Milton P. Siegel.* Online, available at: www.population-security.org/29-APP3.html (accessed 22 August 2008).

Munck, Ronaldo (2002) 'Global civil society: myths and prospects'. *Voluntas* 13: 349–61.

Näth, Marie-Luise (1998) 'The position of the ROC in international organisations: problems and prospects'. In Näth, Marie-Luise (ed.) *The Republic of China on Taiwan in International Politics.* Frankfurt: Peter Lang.

Natsios, Andrew S. (1996) 'NGOs and the UN system in complex humanitarian emergencies: conflict or cooperation?' In Weiss, Thomas G. and Gordenker, Leon (eds) *NGOs, the UN, and Global Governance.* Boulder: Lynne Rienner.

Natsios, Andrew S. (1997) *U.S. Foreign Policy and the Four Horsemen of the Apocalypse: Humanitarian Relief in Complex Emergencies.* The Washington papers/170. Westport: Praeger.

Nederveen Pieterse, Jan (ed.) (1998) *World Orders in the Making: Humanitarian Intervention and beyond.* London: Macmillan.

New York Times (31 March 2004) 'Dominica: Taiwan severs ties'.

NGO Affairs Committee (2006) *Taiwan NGOs Reaching out to the World.* Taipei: NGO Affairs Committee, Ministry of Foreign Affairs, Republic of China (Taiwan).

Ngo, Tak-wing (1995) 'Business encirclement of politics: government-business relations across the Taiwan Strait'. *China Information* 10: 1–18.

Niou, Emerson M. S. (1995) 'An evaluation of the Republic of China's foreign policy alternatives'. In Cheng, Tun-jen and Huang, Chi (eds) *Inherited Rivalry: Conflict across the Taiwan Straits.* Boulder: Lynne Rienner.

Nozick, Robert (1974) *Anarchy, State, and Utopia.* New York: Basic Books.

Nyasa Times (22 January 2008) 'Taiwanese eviction can affect up to 50,000 patients in the Mzuzu area'. Online, available at: http://wellsforzoe.wordpress.com/2008/

01/22/tiawanese-eviction-can-affect-up-to-50000-patients-in-the-mzuzu-area/ (accessed 27 August 2008).

Nye, Joseph S. Jr and Donahue, John D. (eds) (2000) *Governance in a Globalizing World*. Washington, DC: Brookings Institution.

OECD (1978) *Recommendation on Terms and Conditions of Aid*. Online, available at: www.oecd.org/document/59/0,2340,en_2649_34447_31427515_1_1_1_1,00.html (accessed 15 July 2006).

OECD (2001) 'Working Party on Statistics. Is it ODA?' *Note by the Secretariat*. DCD/DAC/STAT(2001)8. Online, available at: http://72.14.203.104/search?q=cache:opy8aC7gAPsJ:www.oecd.org/dataoecd/21/21/34086975.pdf+oecd+should+be+recorded,+but+not+as+development+assistance&hl=en&gl=hk&ct=clnk&cd=1 (accessed 15 July 2006).

OECD (2003) *DAC List of ODA Recipients as at 1 January 2003*. Online, available at: www.oecd.org/dataoecd/35/9/2488552.pdf (accessed 27 April 2005).

OECD (2004) DAC Working Party on Aid Effectiveness and Donor Practices. *Room Document 6*. Online, available at: www.oecd.org/dataoecd/10/20/29734886.pdf (accessed 15 July 2006).

OECD (2005) *DAC List of ODA Recipients as at 1 January 2005*. Online, available at: www.oecd.org/document/45/0,2340,en_2649_34447_2093101_1_1_1_1,00.html (accessed 27 April 2005).

OECD (2008a) *Net Official Development Assistance in 2007: Preliminary Data for 2007*. Online, available at: www.oecd.org/dataoecd/27/55/40381862.pdf (accessed 30 July 2008).

OECD (2008b) 'Debt relief is down: other ODA rises slightly'. Online, available at: www.oecd.org/document/8/0,3343,en_2649_33721_40381960_1_1_1_1,00.html (accessed 2 August 2008).

OECD/DAC (2006) Development Assistance Committee (DAC). Network on Governance (GOVNET). *Draft Principles for Donor Action in Anti-corruption*. Paris: OECD.

OECD/WHO/DAC (2003) DAC Guidelines and Reference Series. *Poverty and Health*. Paris: OECD.

Office of the President, Republic of China (Taiwan) (2006) *President Chen's Remarks at the Videoconference with Prominent European Opinion Leaders in Geneva*. Online, available at: www.gio.gov.tw/taiwan-website/4-oa/20060519/2006051901.html (accessed 25 July 2006).

O'Hanlon, Michael and Singer, P. W. (2004) 'The humanitarian transformation: expanding global intervention capacity'. *Survival* 46: 77–100.

Omoruyi, Leslie O. (2001) *Contending Theories on Development Aid: Post-Cold War Evidence from Africa*. Aldershot: Ashgate.

Permanent Mission of the Peoples' Republic of China to the United Nations Office at Geneva and other international organisations in Switzerland (2003) 'Facts on Taiwanese separatists' "WHO gamble" and cooperation and exchanges on SARS battle across the Taiwan Strait'. 15 May 2003. Online, available at: www.china-un.ch/eng/48748.html (accessed 13 June 2006).

Personal communication from a WHO officer, Geneva, 16 June 2003.

Personal communication from a WHO officer, Geneva, 17 June 2003.

Personal communication from a WHO officer, Geneva, 18 June 2003.

Personal communication from a former executive of Médecins du Monde, Paris, 23 June 2003.

Peters, Guy B. (1988) 'Introduction'. In Campbell, Colin and Peters, Guy B. (eds) *Organizing Governance, Governing Organizations.* Pittsburgh: University of Pittsburgh Press.

Peters, Guy B. (1996) *The Future of Governing: Four Emerging Models.* Lawrence: University Press of Kansas.

Peters, Guy B. (2002a) 'The changing nature of public administration: from easy answers to hard questions'. *Asian Journal of Public Administration* 24: 153–83.

Peters, Guy B. (2002b) 'The politics of tool choice'. In Salamon, Lester M. (ed.) *The Tools of Government: a Guide to the New Governance.* Oxford: Oxford University Press.

Peters, Guy B. and Pierre, Jon (2003) 'Introduction: the role of public administration in governing'. In Peters, Guy B. and Pierre, Jon (eds) *Handbook of Public Administration.* London: Sage.

Peters, Guy B. and van Nispen, Frans K. M. (1998) 'Prologue'. In Peters, Guy B. and van Nispen, Frans K. M. (eds) *Public Policy Instruments: Evaluating the Tools of Public Administration.* Northampton: Edward Elgar.

Pierre, Jon and Peters, Guy B. (2000) *Governance, Politics and the State.* London: Macmillan.

Pierre, Jon and Peters, Guy B. (2005) *Governing Complex Societies: Trajectories and Scenarios.* Basingstoke: Palgrave Macmillan.

Ramsbotham, Oliver and Woodhouse, Tom (1996) *Humanitarian Intervention in Contemporary Conflict.* Cambridge: Polity Press.

Reliefweb (29 November 1999) *Taiwan Earthquake Fact Sheet #6.* Online, available at: wwww.reliefweb.int/rw/rwb.nsf/AllDocsByUNID/ca2f6d2ace2d2b69c12567fc0030bee a (accessed 13 June 2006).

Reno, William (1998) *Warlord Politics and African States.* Boulder: Lynne Rienner.

Reporters without Borders (22 May 2008) 'RSF calls for "balance in matters of news and information" in support of Taiwanese journalists'. Online, available at: www.ifex.org/en/content/view/full/93956 (accessed 23 August 2008).

Republic of China Yearbook Taiwan (2002) *Foreign Relations: People's Diplomacy.* Online, available at: www.gio.gov.tw/taiwan-website/5-gp/yearbook/2002/chpt09–1.htm (accessed 20 August 2006).

Rigger, Shelley (1996) 'Mobilisational authoritarianism and political opposition in Taiwan'. In Rodan, Garry (ed.) *Political Oppositions in Industrialising Asia.* London: Routledge.

Rollet, Vincent (2005) 'Taiwanese NGOs and HIV/Aids: from the national to the transnational'. *China Perspectives* 60. Online, available at: http://chinaperspectives.revues.org/document498.html (accessed 22 August 2008).

Rosenau, James N. (1992) 'Governance, order and change in world politics'. In Rosenau, James N. and Czempiel Ernst-Otto (eds) *Governance without Government: Order and Change in World Politics.* Cambridge: Cambridge University Press.

Rotary International (2001) 'First Taiwanese elected vice president of international business organisation'. *Press Release from Rotary International.* 14 July 2001. Online, available at: www.roc-taiwan.org/chicago/press/20010714/2001071401.html (accessed 24 April 2005).

Rufin, Jean-Christophe (1993) 'The paradoxes of armed protection'. In Jean, François (ed.) *Life, Death and Aid: the Médecins Sans Frontières Report on World Crisis Intervention.* London: Routledge.

Salamon, Lester M. (ed.) (2002) *The Tools of Government: a Guide to the New Governance.* Oxford: Oxford University Press.

Schmidt, Vivien (2006) 'Institutionalism'. In Hay, Colin, Lister, Michael and Marsh, David (eds) *The State: Theories and Issues*. Basingstoke: Palgrave Macmillan.

Schmitt, Carl (1996) *The Concept of the Political*, trans. J Harvey Lomax. Chicago: University of Chicago Press.

Schnabel, Albrecht and Thakur, Ramesh (eds) (2000) *Kosovo and the Challenge of Humanitarian Intervention: Selective Indignation, Collective Action and International Citizenship*. Tokyo: United Nations University Press.

Scholte, Jan A. (2000) *Globalization: a Critical Introduction*. Basingstoke: Macmillan Press.

Sedemund, Jens (2008) 'Taiwan and OECD'. E-mail (19 August 2008).

Shaw, Yu-ming (1979) 'Modern history of Taiwan: an interpretative account'. In Chiu, Hungdah (ed.) *China and the Taiwan Issue*. New York: Praeger.

Sheng, Emile C. J. (2002) 'Cross-Strait relations and public opinion on Taiwan'. *Issues and Studies* 38: 17–46.

Siddiqi, Javed (1995) *World Health and World Politics*. London: Hurst.

Sinn, Elizabeth (1989) *Power and Charity: the Early History of the Tung Wah Hospital*. Hong Kong: Oxford University Press.

Smillie, Ian (1997) 'NGOs and development assistance: a change of mind-set?' *Third World Quarterly* 18: 563–77.

Smith, Edwin M. and Weiss, Thomas G. (1997) 'UN task-sharing: towards or away from global governance?' *Third World Quarterly* 18: 595–619.

Sohn, Louis B. (1996) 'Taiwan's option of becoming a permanent observer'. In Henckaerts, Jean-Marie (ed.) *The International Status of Taiwan in the New World Order: Legal and Political Considerations*. London: Kluwer Law International.

Sorensen, Georg (2006) 'The transformation of the state'. In Hay, Colin, Lister, Michael and Marsh, David (eds) *The State: Theories and Issues*. Basingstoke: Palgrave Macmillan.

South China Morning Post (2 April 2005) 'Taipei wary of offer to help it join health body'.

South China Morning Post (2 August 2005) 'Taipei seeks diplomatic role with NGO grouping'.

Sovereign Order of Malta (2008) *Bilateral Relations with Countries*. Online, available at: www.orderofmalta.org/site/attdiplomatica.asp?idlingua=5 (accessed 31 August 2008).

Straits Times (8 November 2005) 'Chen brushes off criticism of aid disclosure'.

Sutter, Robert (1999) 'Taipei's struggle for influence over U.S. policy'. In Chao, Chien-min and Clark, Cal (eds) *The ROC on the Threshold of the 21st Century: a Paradigm Reexamined*. Baltimore: University of Maryland School of Law.

Sybesma-Knol, Neri (1996) 'The United Nations framework for the participation of observers'. In Henckaerts, Jean-Marie (ed.) *The International Status of Taiwan in the New World Order: Legal and Political Considerations*. London: Kluwer Law International.

Taipei Journal (2 February 2001) 'Christians contribute to Taiwan society'. Online, available at: www.taiwanheadlines.gov.tw/20010208/20010206f3.html (accessed 7 March 2005).

Taipei Times (25 September 1999) 'Taipei accuses China of exploiting quake'. Online, available at: www.taipeitimes.com/News/front/archives/1999/09/25/3912 (accessed 22 August 2008).

Taipei Times (18 August 2000) 'NGO's give Taiwan vital world role'. Online, available at: www.taipeitimes.com/News/editorials/archives/2000/08/18/48296 (accessed 22 August 2008).

Taipei Times (3 October 2000) 'NGO group makes plea'. Online, available at: www.taipeitimes.com/News/local/archives/2000/10/03/55819 (accessed 22 August 2008).

Taipei Times (31 October 2000) 'Health officials plan to protest WHO oversight'. Online, available at: www.taipeitimes.com/News/local/archives/2000/10/31/59305 (accessed 22 August 2008).

Taipei Times (1 November 2000) 'Taiwan plans to sponsor UN AIDS programs'. Online, available at: www.taipeitimes.com/News/local/archives/2000/11/01/59473 (accessed 22 August 2008).

Taipei Times (21 December 2000) 'NGOs seek cooperation with government'. Online, available at: www.taipeitimes.com/News/local/archives/2000/12/21/66388 (accessed 22 August 2008).

Taipei Times (16 June 2001) 'The promises and pitfalls of NGOs'. Online, available at: www.taipeitimes.com/News/editorials/archives/2001/06/16/90247 (accessed 22 August 2008).

Taipei Times (13 April 2002) 'DPP members want 'Taiwan' on WHO bid'. Online, available at: www.taipeitimes.com/News/taiwan/archives/2002/04/13/131665 (accessed 22 August 2008).

Taipei Times (13 May 2002) 'Bid for WHO luring hundreds to Geneva'. Online, available at: www.taipeitimes.com/News/front/archives/2002/05/13/135813/print (accessed 22 August 2008).

Taipei Times (16 May 2002) 'Taiwan expects to give US$1m to WHO fund'. Online, available at: www.taipeitimes.com/News/front/archives/2002/05/16/136218 (accessed 22 August 2008).

Taipei Times (19 May 2003a) 'Leading medical organizations support new bid'. Online, available at: www.taipeitimes.com/News/taiwan/archives/2003/05/19/211161 (accessed 22 August 2008).

Taipei Times (19 May 2003b) 'Taiwan makes progress at WHO'. Online, available at: www.taipeitimes.com/News/front/archives/2003/05/19/211140 (accessed 22 August 2008).

Taipei Times (20 May 2003) 'WHO shoots down Assembly entry bid'. Online, available at: www.taipeitimes.com/News/front/archives/2003/05/20/2003051820 (accessed 22 August 2008).

Taipei Times (21 May 2003) 'No voice for Taiwan at WHO meet'. Online, available at: www.taipeitimes.com/News/front/archives/2003/05/21/2003051963 (accessed 22 August 2008).

Taipei Times (7 July 2003) 'Tibetan association leader says relations markedly improved'. Online, available at: www.taipeitimes.com/News/taiwan/archives/2003/07/07/2003058381 (accessed 22 August 2008).

Taipei Times (10 May 2004) 'The myth of the 'apolitical' WTO'. Online, available at: www.taipeitimes.com/News/editorials/archives/2004/05/10/2003154901 (accessed 22 August 2008).

Taipei Times (17 May 2004a) 'US could back Taiwan WHO bid'. Online, available at: www.taipeitimes.com/News/taiwan/archives/2004/05/17/2003155829 (accessed 22 August 2008).

Taipei Times (17 May 2004b) 'WHA: Taiwan pins its hopes on allies'. Online, available at: www.taipeitimes.com/News/front/archives/2004/05/17/2003155813 (accessed 22 August 2008).

Taipei Times (16 June 2004) 'US bill supporting WHA bid now law'. Online, available at: www.taipeitimes.com/News/taiwan/archives/2004/06/16/2003175244 (accessed 22 August 2008).

Taipei Times (14 February 2005) 'International health NGO to host meeting in Taipei'. Online, available at: www.taipeitimes.com/News/taiwan/archives/2005/02/14/2003223006 (accessed 22 August 2008).

Taipei Times (24 February 2005) 'Ministry says food donation to Iraq was sold as fodder'. Online, available at: www.taipeitimes.com/News/taiwan/archives/2005/02/24/2003224365 (accessed 22 August 2008).

Taipei Times (15 January 2008) 'Malawi, Taiwan end 42-year relations'. Online, available at: www.taipeitimes.com/News/front/archives/2008/01/15/2003397305 (accessed 22 August 2008).

Taipei Times (4 April 2008) 'No WHA observer status anytime soon'. Online, available at: www.taipeitimes.com/News/taiwan/archives/2008/04/04/2003408245 (accessed 1 September 2008).

Taiwan Center for Disease Control (CDC) (2005) *Taiwan's Participation in the WHO is Vital for Fighting the Threat of Avian Flu*. Online, available at: www.mofa.gov.tw/public/Attachment/51116129071.doc (accessed 25 August 2008).

Taiwan Department of Health (2003) International Cooperation Bureau. *A Study on International Medical Assistance and Cooperation by the Government and Private Organizations in Taiwan between 1996 and 2002*. Unpublished.

Taiwan Department of Health (undated) *SARS and China's Absurd Claims*. (Courtesy of a senior WHO officer).

Taiwan Government (2008) *Taiwan's WHO Bid for 2008*. Online, available at: http://english.www.gov.tw/public/Data/842517183471.pdf (accessed 3 August 2008).

Taiwan Government Information Office (2004) *Rebuttal to PRC Arguments against Inviting Taiwan to Participate in the WHO*. Online, available at: www.gio.gov.tw/taiwan-website/5-gp/join_who/2004/who16.htm (accessed 23 August 2008).

Taiwan Government Information Office (14 May 2004) *Media Background Note: Taiwanese People Hope for Health with Dignity*. Online, available at: www.gio.gov.tw/taiwan-website/5-gp/join_who/2004/who191.htm (accessed 19 July 2008).

Taiwan Headlines (22 November 1999) 'Tzu-Chi plans global relief network'. Online, available at: www.taiwanheadlines.gov.tw/19991122/19991122s6.html (accessed 3 August 2006).

Taiwan Headlines (11 December 2001) 'The ROC's humanitarian relief program for Afghan refugees'. Online, available at: www.roc-taiwan.org.uk/taiwan/5-gp/relief/help_41.htm (accessed 26 August 2006).

Taiwan International Cooperation and Development Fund (TaiwanICDF) (2004) *Annual Report 2003*. Taipei: ICDF-TAIWAN.

Taiwan International Cooperation and Development Fund (TaiwanICDF) (2007) *Annual Report 2006*. Taipei: ICDF-TAIWAN. Online, available at: www.icdf.org.tw/english/e_pub_anual_contect.asp?pid=163 (accessed 2 September 2008).

Taiwan International Cooperation and Development Fund (TaiwanICDF) (2008) *Annual Report 2007*. Taipei: ICDF-TAIWAN. Online, available at: www.icdf.org.tw/english/e_pub_anual_contect.asp?pid=170 (accessed 19 August 2008).

Taiwan International Health Action (TaiwanIHA) (2007a) 'About TaiwanIHA'. Online, available at: www.taiwaniha.org.tw/eaboutus.html (accessed 25 August 2008).

Taiwan International Health Action (TaiwanIHA) (2007b) *Passion and Care: 2000–2006 the Story of Taiwan's Global Health Humanitarian Aid*. Taipei: Taiwan International Health Action (TaiwanIHA). Online, available at: www.taiwaniha.org.tw/publish/passion/passion.pdf (accessed 2 August 2008).

Taiwan International Medical Alliance (2003) 'What's TIMA?' Online, available at: www.tima.org.tw/English_view/What%27s%20TIMA.html (accessed 20 August 2006).

Taiwan International Medical Alliance (2004) *Introduction of Taiwan Nongovernmental Organizations with International Health Cooperation Activities*. Taipei: Taiwan International Medical Alliance.

Taiwan Ministry of Foreign Affairs (2005a). *Concept Paper #1: The Legality of Taiwan's Participation in the WHA as an Observer in the Capacity of Health Entity*. Online, available at: www.mofa.gov.tw/public/Attachment/54291202158.pdf (accessed 23 August 2008).

Taiwan Ministry of Foreign Affairs (2005b). *Concept Paper #2. The Global Health Imperatives for Granting Taiwan WHA Observership*. Online, available at: www.mofa.gov.tw/public/Attachment/471315462471.pdf (accessed 23 August 2008).

Taiwan Ministry of Foreign Affairs (2006). 'TaiwanIHA to sponsor 28th World Congress of Internal Medicine'. Online, available at: www.mofa.gov.tw/webapp/fp.asp?xItem=23351&ctNode=1014 (accessed 2 September 2008).

Taiwan Ministry of Foreign Affairs (undated) *Concept Paper #3. Rebuttal to PRC Arguments against Inviting Taiwan as an Observer to the WHA*. Online, available at: www.mofa.gov.tw/webapp/public/Attachment/54291231171.pdf (accessed 13 June 2006).

Taiwan News (23 September 1999a) 'MAC considering China's offer of assistance for quake victims'.

Taiwan News (23 September 1999b) 'China's Red Cross offers assistance'.

Taiwan News (11 June 2002) 'MOFA lauds achievements of local NGOs'.

Taiwan Philanthropy Information Center (2004) 'World Vision Taiwan celebrates its 40th Anniversary'. Online, available at: www.tpic.org.tw/EPhilNews/show_news.asp?ENEWSID=4087 (accessed 7 March 2005).

Taiwan Review (30 November 2006) 'What really counts'. Online, available at: http://taiwanreview.nat.gov.tw/ct.asp?CtNode=119&xItem=23510 (accessed 2 August 2008).

Taiwan Thinktank (2006) *Public Survey Presentation and Forum on the Taiwan Public's View of the President's Visits and Taiwan's Foreign Relations*. Online, available at: www.taiwanthinktank.org/ttt/servlet/OpenBlock?Template=Article&lan=en&category_id=58&article_id=651&BlockSet= (accessed 18 July 2008).

Taiwan Thinktank (2007a) *Cross-Strait Relations: Two Years after the Pass of China's Anti-Secession Law*. Online, available at: www.taiwanthinktank.org/ttt/attachment/article_731_attach3.pdf (accessed 19 August 2008).

Taiwan Thinktank (2007b) *Taiwan's UN Bid and Foreign Relations*. Online, available at: www.taiwanthinktank.org/ttt/attachment/article_696_attach1.pdf (accessed 19 August 2008).

Taiwan Thinktank (2008) *Taiwan's UN Participation and Foreign Relations*. Online, available at: www.taiwanthinktank.org/ttt/attachment/article_871_attach4.pdf (accessed 19 August 2008).

Taiwanese Young Professionals Association of Quebec (2007) *Taiwan's WHO Membership Bid for 2007*. Online, available at: www.typaq.ca/news-events/news/detailnews/?tx_ttnews%5Btt_news%5D=1&tx_ttnews%5BbackPid%5D=2&cHash=78a3a16ff (accessed 3 August 2008).

Tang, James T. H. (1993) 'Hong Kong's International Status'. *Pacific Review* 6: 205–15.

Taylor, Rupert (2002) 'Interpreting global civil society'. *Voluntas* 13: 339–47.

Teklehaimanot, Awash (2003) *Report on Malaria Mission to São Tomé and Príncipe*. Online, available at: www.earthinstitute.columbia.edu/gsd/STP/documents/Report-MalariaMssionOct03.pdf (accessed 13 July 2006).

Telephone interview with Yan-di Chang, 25 October 2004.

Terry, Fiona (2002) *Condemned to Repeat? The Paradox of Humanitarian Action*. Ithaca: Cornell University Press.

Tesón, Fernando R (1996) *Humanitarian Intervention: an Inquiry into Law and Morality*. 2nd edn. Irvington-On-Hudson: Transnational.

Thomas, Caroline and Weber, Martin (2004) 'The politics of global health governance: whatever happened to 'health for all by the year 2000'?' *Global Governance* 10: 187–205.

Thynne, Ian (2000) 'The state and governance: issues and challenges in perspective'. *International Review of Administrative Sciences* 66: 227–40.

Tilly, Charles (1985) 'War making and state making as organised crime'. In Evans, Peter B., Rueschemeyer, Dietrich and Skocpol, Theda (eds) *Bringing the State back in*. Cambridge: Cambridge University Press.

Timesonline (3 July 2006) 'It kept quiet about Sars – now has China been caught out over bird flu?' Online, available at: www.timesonline.co.uk/article/0,,20909–2253760,00.html (accessed 21 August 2006).

Tkacik, John J (29 April 2004) 'Offer real support, not excuses, for Taiwan's WHO bid'. *Executive Memorandum #927*. The Heritage Foundation. Online, available at: www.heritage.org/Research/AsiaandthePacific/em927.cfm (accessed 23 July 2004).

Tsai, Eddy (1999) 'Why the Republic of China should be included in WHO'. *The Lancet* 354: 2157.

Tsang, Steve (1999) 'Transforming a party state into a democracy'. In Tsang, Steve and Tien, Hung-mao (eds) *Democratization in Taiwan: Implications for China*. Hong Kong: Hong Kong University Press.

Tubilewicz, Czes (2001) 'Taiwan's Balkan option: a new chapter in Republic of China "dollar diplomacy"'. *Diplomacy and Statecraft* 12: 161–84.

Tzu Chi (1997) 'Liberian First Lady visits Tzuchi Taipei branch office'. Online, available at: http://taipei.tzuchi.org.tw/tzquart/97winter/qw97–22.htm (accessed 20 August 2006).

Tzu Chi (1999) 'Refugee camps in Albania receive 4,600 pounds of medicine'. Online, available at: http://taipei.tzuchi.org.tw/tzquart/99summer/qs99–22.htm (accessed 20 August 2006).

Tzu Chi (2000) *Enveloping the World with Great Love. The Tzu-chi International Relief Effort 1991–2000*. Online, available at: http://taipei.tzuchi.org.tw/tzquart/book/book2/4.htm (accessed 24 June 2006).

Tzu Chi News (1 June 2003) 'Rice aid to Indonesia'. Online, available at: www.tzuchi.org/global/news/articles/20030601.html (accessed 22 August 2006).

Tzu Chi News (15 December 2003) 'Tzu Chi recognized as an United Nations Non-Govermental Organization (NGO)'. Online, available at: www.tzuchi.org/Global/news/articles/20031215.html (accessed 26 June 2006).

Tzu Chi News (18 July 2004) 'Nine ambassadors and representatives from Africa visit Tzu Chi'. Online, available at: www.tzuchi.org/global/news/articles/20040718.html (accessed 4 March 2005).

UNAIDS (undated) 'About UNAIDS'. Online, available at: www.unaids.org/en/about+unaids/what+is+unaids.asp (accessed 19 February 2005).

UNICEF (2003) *Annual Report 2003*. Online, available at: www.unicef.org/publications/files/unicef_eng_final.pdf (accessed 24 April 2005).

UNICEF (2006a) *Expanding Immunization Coverage*. Online, available at: www.unicef.org/immunization/index_coverage.html (accessed 15 July 2006).

UNICEF (2006b) 'Under the moonlight, UNICEF's mobile cinema helps prevent malaria in Sao Tome'. Online, available at: www.unicef.org/infobycountry/stp_31755.html (accessed 15 July 2006).

UNICEF (undated) *Immunization: Introduction.* Online, available at: www.unicef.org/immunization/index.html (accessed 24 April 2005).

Union of International Associations (ed.) (2004) *Yearbook of International Organisations 2003/2004.* (vol. 5). München: K.G.Saur.

Union of International Associations (ed.) (2007) *Yearbook of International Organisations: Guide to Global and Civil Society Networks, Edition 44, 2007/2008. Volume 5: Statistics, Visualizations and Patterns.* München: K.G.Saur.

United Kingdom Parliament (2000) *House of Commons Hansard Debates for 2 Feb 2000* (pt5). Online, available at: www.parliament.the-stationery-office.co.uk/pa/cm199900/cmhansrd/vo000202/halltext/00202h05.htm (accessed 24 July 2004).

United Nations (1993) *Request for the Inclusion of a Supplementary Item in the Agenda of the 48th Session, Consideration of the Exceptional Situation of the Republic of China in Taiwan in the International Context, based on the Principle of Universality and in accordance with the Established Model of Parallel Representation of Divided Countries at the United Nations.* U.N. Doc. A/48/191 (9 August 1993).

United Nations (2005) *Millennium Development Goals: Progress Chart.* Online, available at: http://72.14.203.104/search?q=cache:EJfqhNCck44J:www.un.org/millenniumgoals/mdg_chart_sept.pdf+kofi+annan+millennium+progress+report&hl=en&gl=hk&ct=clnk&cd=1 (accessed 15 July 2006).

United Nations Department of Public Information (1999) *Press Release SC/6648.* 'UNPREDEP's mandate not renewed beyond 28 February 1999 as Council does not adopt draft on six-month extension due to veto by China'. Online, available at: www.un.org/Depts/dpko/dpko/co_mission/unpred_r.htm (accessed 14 July 2006).

United Nations General Assembly (2000) *United Nations Millennium Declaration.* A/55/L.2. Online, available at: www.un.org/millennium/declaration/ares552e.htm (accessed 30 June 2006).

Unrepresented Nations and Peoples Organization (undated) *Introduction.* Online, available at: www.unpo.org/introduction.php (accessed 19 August 2006).

Vale, Peter (1997) 'South Africa and Taiwan: pariahs, international redemption, and global change'. In Yang, Maysing H. (ed.) *Taiwan's Expanding Role in the International Arena.* London: M.E. Sharpe.

Vedung, Evert (1998) 'Policy instruments: typologies and theories'. In Bemelmans-Videc, Marie-Louise, Rist, Ray C. and Vedung, Evert (eds) *Carrots, Sticks and Sermons: Policy Instruments and their Evaluation.* New Brunswick: Transaction.

Vogel, David (2005) *The Market for Virtue: The Potential and Limits of Corporate Social Responsibility.* Washington, DC: Brookings Institution Press.

Waltz, Kenneth (1979) *Theory of International Politics.* New York: Addison-Wesley.

Wang, James C. F. (1994) *Comparative Asian Politics: Power, Policy, and Change.* Englewood Cliffs: Prentice Hall.

Wang Kuo-chang (1984) *United Nations Voting on Chinese Representation: an Analysis of General Assembly Roll-calls 1950–1971.* Taipei: Institute of American Culture, Academia Sinica.

Wang, Qingxin Ken (2000) 'Taiwanese NGOs and the prospect of national reunification in the Taiwan Strait'. *Australian Journal of International Affairs* 54: 111–24.

Waterman, Peter (1999) 'Activists beyond borders – and theorists within them'. *Transnational Associations* 51: 39–40.

Weber, Max (1978) *Economy and Society*. New York: Bedminster.

Weiss, Thomas G. and Gordenker, Leon (1996) 'Pluralizing global governance: analytical approaches and dimensions'. In Weiss, Thomas G. and Gordenker, Leon (eds) *NGOs, the UN, and Global Governance*. Boulder: Lynne Rienner.

Weiss, Thomas and Minear, Larry (eds) (1993) *Humanitarianism across Borders: Sustaining Civilians in Times of War*. Boulder: Lynne Rienner.

Wendt, Alexander (1999) *Social Theory of International Politics*. Cambridge: Cambridge University Press.

Whitehead, Margaret, Dahlgren, Göran, and Evans, Timothy (2001) 'Equity and health sector reforms: can low-income countries escape the medical poverty trap?' *The Lancet* 358: 833–6.

Woodward, D. and Smith, R. D. (2003) 'Global public goods and health: concepts and issues'. In Smith, R. D., Beaglehole, R., Woodward, D. and Drager, N. (eds) *Global Public Goods for Health: Health, Economic and Public Health Perspectives*. Oxford: Oxford University Press.

World Bank (2004) *Annual Report 2004*. Online, available at: www.worldbank.org/annualreport/2004/pdf/thematic_perspectives.pdf (accessed 24 April 2005).

World Bank (2005) *Annual Report 2005*. Online, available at: http://siteresources.worldbank.org/INTANNREP2K5/Resources/51563_English.pdf (accessed 19 August 2008).

World Bank (undated) *Measuring Results*. Online, available at: http://web.worldbank.org/WBSITE/EXTERNAL/PROJECTS/0,,contentMDK:20120723~menuPK:41393~pagePK:41367~piPK:51533~theSitePK:40941,00.html (accessed 24 April 2005).

World Health Organization (1973) WHA 25.1. *Handbook of Resolutions and Decisions of the World Health Assembly and the Executive Board. Volume I 1948–1972*. Geneva: World Health Organization.

World Health Organization (1978) *Memorandum of Understanding on the Administrative and Technical Structures of the Special Programme for Research and Training in Tropical Diseases*. TDR/CP/78.5/Rev.2006. Online, available at: www.who.int/tdr/about/governance/basic-documents/mou.htm (accessed 22 August 2006).

World Health Organization (1997) *Fiftieth World Health Assembly. Geneva, 5–14 May 1997. Verbatim Records of Plenary Meetings*. WHA50/1997/REC/2. Geneva: World Health Organization.

World Health Organization (1998a) 'Health-for-all policy for the twenty-first century'. Agenda item 19. WHA51.7. 16 May 1998. Online, available at: www.who.int/archives/hfa/ear7.pdf (accessed 28 July 2004).

World Health Organization (1998b) 'Enterovirus outbreak in Taiwan, China'. 16 June 1998. Online, available at: www.who.int/disease-outbreak-news/n1998/jun/n16june1998.html (accessed 27 July 2004).

World Health Organization (2000a). *53rd World Health Assembly. Agenda Item 17. Collaboration within the United Nations System and with other Intergovernmental Organizations. Aligning the Participation of Palestine in the World Health Organization with its Participation in the United Nations. Annex*. Draft A53/40 (19 May 2000). Geneva: World Health Organization. Online, available at: http://ftp.who.int/gb/archive/pdf_files/WHA53/ea40.pdf (accessed 19 August 2008).

World Health Organization (2000b) *The World Health Report 2000. Health Systems: Improving Performance*. Geneva: World Health Organization.

World Health Organization (2001a) *Principles Governing Relations between the World Health Organisation and Non-governmental Organisations*. WHO. Basic documents. Geneva: World Health Organization.

World Health Organization (2001b) *Guidelines for Interaction with Commercial Enterprises to Achieve Health Outcomes.* Executive Board, 107th session, 30 November 2000. Provisional agenda item 8.3. EB 107/20 Annex. Geneva: World Health Organization.

World Health Organization (2002a) Civil society initiative. *WHO and Civil Society: Linking for Better Health.* WHO/CSI/2002/DP1. Geneva: World Health Organization.

World Health Organization (2002b) Civil society initiative. *Understanding Civil Society: Issues for WHO. Discussion Paper No 2.* February 2002. CSI/2002/DP2. Geneva: World Health Organization.

World Health Organization (2002c) Civil society initiative. *Review Report. WHO's Interactions with Civil Society and Nongovernmental Organizations.* WHO/CSI/2002/WP6. Geneva: World Health Organization.

World Health Organization (2002d) *Improving Health Outcomes of the Poor. The Report of Working Group 5 of the Commission on Macroeconomics and Health.* Geneva: World Health Organization.

World Health Organization (2003a) Fifty-sixth World Health Assembly. *Provisional Agenda Item 21.* 14 April 2003. A56/46. Geneva: World Health Organization.

World Health Organization (2003b) Executive Board, 111th session, 5 February 2003. EB111/SR/10. Geneva: World Health Organization.

World Health Organization (2003c) *Severe Acute Respiratory Syndrome-Taiwan, China. Summary of Events, 14 March-16 May 2003.* Amended 16 May 2003. Courtesy of WHO's Press Office. Geneva: World Health Organization.

World Health Organization (2004a) Fifty-seventh World Health Assembly. Geneva 17–22 May 2004. *Summary Records of Committees. Reports of Committees.* WHA57/2004/REC/3. Geneva: World Health Organization.

World Health Organization (2004b) *Proposed Programme Budget 2006–2007.* EB115/INF.DOC./4. 23 December 2004. Online, available at: www.who.int/gb/e/e_eb115.html (accessed 23 June 2006).

World Health Organization (2004c) WHA57/2004/REC/2. Fifty-seventh World Health Assembly. *Verbatim Records of Plenary Meetings and List of Participants.* Geneva, 17–22 May 2004. Geneva: World Health Organization.

World Health Organization (2006a) *Global Outbreak Alert and Response Network.* Online, available at: www.who.int/csr/outbreaknetwork/en/ (accessed 20 August 2006).

World Health Organization (2006b) *Polio Eradication Initiative: Global 2005 Annual Report.* Geneva: World Health Organization.

World Health Organization (2007) *Basic Documents.* 46th edn. Including amendments adopted up to 31 December 2006. Geneva: World Health Organization. Online, available at: www.who.int/gb/bd/PDF/bd46/e-bd46.pdf (accessed 31 August 2008).

World Health Organization (undated) 'Health for all in the 21st century'. Online, available at: www.who.int/archives/hfa/history.htm (accessed 28 July 2004).

World Health Organization/CMH Support Unit (2003) *Investing in Health: a Summary of the Findings of the Commission on Macroeconomics and Health.* Geneva: World Health Organization.

World Medical Association (1997) 'Chinese doctors join the World Medical Association'. *Press release.* 14 November 1997. Online, available at: www.wma.net/e/press/1997_7.htm (accessed 15 March 2006).

World Vision (undated) *Core Values.* Online, available at: www.worldvision.org.tw/english/wv-value.html (accessed 7 March 2005).

Wu, Jaushieh Joseph (1995) *Taiwan's Democratization: Forces behind the New Momentum.* Hong Kong: Oxford University Press.

Wu, Shuh-min (2004) Interview with Dr Shuh-min Wu, President, Foundation of Medical Professionals Alliance in Taiwan, Taipei, 23 September 2004.

Wu, Yu-shan (2000) 'Theorizing on relations across the Taiwan Strait: nine contending approaches'. *Journal of Contemporary China* 9: 407–28.

Young, Oran R. (2005) 'Regime theory and the quest for global governance'. In Ba, Alice D. and Hoffmann, Matthew J. (eds) *Contending Perspectives on Global Governance: Coherence, Contestation and World Order*. London: Routledge.

Yu, J. K.-L., Chen, C., Chang, W., Juma, H. and Chang, C. (2005) 'Fingerprint identification of AIDS patients on ART'. *Lancet* 365: 1466.

Yu, J. K.-L., Chen, C. C., Wang, K. Y., Chang, C. S., Makombe, S. D., Schouten, E. J. and Harries, A. D. (2007) 'True outcomes for patients on antiretroviral therapy who are "lost to follow-up" in Malawi'. *Bulletin of the World Health Organization* 85: 550–4.

Yu, J. K.-L., Bong, C. N., Chen, S. C. C., Dzimadzi, R., Lu, D. Y., Makombe, S., Schouten, E., Kamoto, K. and Harries, A. (2008) 'Outcomes in HIV-infected patients who develop tuberculosis after starting antiretroviral treatment in Malawi [Short Communication]'. *The International Journal of Tuberculosis and Lung Disease* 12: 692–4.

Index

accountability 97, 108, 135–6, 177
advocacy 21, 27, 119, 127
African countries 130, 136, 158
agencies, specialized 30, 35, 40, 54–5, 58, 81, 101
agenda 26, 42, 53, 64, 66, 69, 77, 96, 102, 119, 157, 176; provisional 62, 68–9
agenda item 68, 70
aid operations 125–6, 133, 140
aid outputs 8, 156, 163, 165; Taiwan's 7, 107
aid programmes, Taiwan's 1, 89, 108, 174
aid recipient countries 125, 142; *see also* recipients
allies 38–9, 70–1, 102, 114, 136, 138–9, 151, 167–9; Taiwan's 68, 70, 137, 172; *see also* diplomatic allies
APEC 40, 92–3, 101, 172
associate members 61, 68–9; obligations of 62
associations 48, 51, 72, 74–5, 122, 145, 163
authoritarianism 44–5

Beijing 36, 38–9, 43, 58, 77, 86, 89–90, 101, 104, 138–40, 145, 147, 160
bilateral aid 118, 140, 152, 160
Brazil 73, 158–9
Burkina-Faso 130, 153

Cairo Declaration 37, 180
CARE-France 123, 130, 133, 140, 149–50, 160
Caritas-Taiwan 111, 117, 124, 133
CCMs (Country-Coordinating Mechanisms) 122
CDC (Center for Disease Control) 85, 87–8, 121, 148
Central Intelligence Agency 83, 154
Chad 39, 123, 130, 132, 134, 149, 154, 160, 165, 170, 174
Chan, Margaret 82, 94, 103, 105, 167
Chi-Chi earthquake 57, 86, 90, 167
Chiang Kai-shek 39, 42, 45, 51
China's Taiwan policy 103
China, representation of 36, 80, 95
Chinese Medical Association 68
Chinese Red Cross 90, 117, 147
Civil Society Initiative (CSI) 22, 27, 63
civil society, global 11, 26, 96
Clinton 43, 157
CoA *see* Council of Agriculture
Cold War 15, 31, 37–8, 81, 135
Commission on Macroeconomics and Health 111, 118, 137, 168
communicable diseases 55, 84, 87–8; *see also* infectious diseases
conflicts 3, 15, 28–31, 41, 94, 101, 172, 176–8
Congressional Taiwan Caucus (CTC) 51
connections, personal 149–50, 173–4
corporatism 46, 48
Council of Agriculture (CoA) 7, 114–15, 125, 130–1, 151
countries: disease-endemic 109, 111; divided 15, 81; donor 7, 107, 114, 152, 161; friendly 75, 108, 110, 115; least developed 157–60; low-income 119, 160; recipient 119, 122, 138, 140, 153, 157, 160; resource-poor 14, 26, 31, 84; sovereign 35, 40
Country-Coordinating Mechanisms (CCMs) 122
CSI *see* Civil Society Initiative
CTC (Congressional Taiwan Caucus) 51

DAC (Development Aid Committee) 118, 121, 140–1, 151, 153, 161, 173

Democratic Pacific Union (DPU) 41, 172
Department of Health (DoH) 58, 66, 71, 114–15, 119, 125, 129, 132, 140, 148, 150–1, 155, 161
Department of International Organizations 114, 119
Department of Public Information (DPI) 133, 163, 174
Development Aid Committee *see* DAC
developmental state 44; strong 5, 43
DIO *see* Department of International Organizations
diplomatic allies 41, 66, 68–9, 80, 82, 100, 119, 138–9, 145, 150, 161, 167, 172–3; *see also* allies
diplomatic isolation 39–42, 48, 174; Taiwan's 51, 146, 156
disasters 28, 30, 34, 75, 86, 114, 119–20, 134, 165, 169–71, 173, 175
disease control 56–8, 83, 85, 87–8, 121
DNDi *see* Drugs for Neglected Diseases initiative
DoH *see* Department of Health
dollar diplomacy 1, 49
DPI *see* Department of Public Information
DPU *see* Democratic Pacific Union
Drugs for Neglected Diseases initiative (DNDi) 121, 128

ECOSOC (Economic and Social Council) 33, 54, 97, 113, 122, 163, 174
enterovirus 57, 85, 88, 90
epidemic outbreaks 28, 31, 53, 65, 84–6, 88, 99; *see also* outbreaks
epidemics 32, 53–5, 57–9, 76, 88–9, 99, 113, 115, 127
Europe 14, 36, 53, 65, 74, 98, 112, 129
exclusion 35, 54–60, 68, 81–3, 89, 98, 102, 166–7; Taiwan's 56, 59, 83, 86, 91

FAPA (Formosan Association for Public Affairs) 51, 68, 75, 96
flu pandemic 76
FMPAT (Foundation of Medical Professionals Alliance in Taiwan) 67, 74, 94, 116, 149
food aid 114–15, 119, 124, 130–1, 157–8, 169, 177–8
Formosan Association for Public Affairs *see* FAPA
Foundation of Medical Professionals Alliance in Taiwan *see* FMPAT

Geneva 4, 30, 59, 66, 74–5, 87, 91, 93, 95, 97–8, 104
Geneva Conventions 28, 30
GHIs *see* Global Health Initiatives
Global Fund 76, 94, 113, 119, 121–2, 128, 130, 140, 148–50, 154–5, 157, 161, 167, 170, 173–4
Global Health Initiatives (GHIs) 121, 123
Global Outbreak Alert and Response Network (GOARN) 65, 85, 87, 91, 98–9, 105, 166
global public goods (GPGs) 27, 97, 159, 177
Global Public–Private Partnerships for Health (GPPHs) 122, 128
Global public–private partnerships *see* GPPPs
Global TB Alliance 121, 128
governance actors 3, 5–6, 35, 61, 80, 91, 107, 112, 141, 165, 176
governance discourses 5, 9, 17
governance elements 3–6, 13, 29, 36, 53, 165–6, 170, 176
governance norms 6, 54, 80, 107, 135, 163, 166, 170, 176; *see also* norms
governance outputs 76, 98, 126, 152
governance processes 2, 6–7, 19, 34, 36, 68, 80, 95, 107, 117–18, 147, 167–8, 176–7
governance systems 4, 6, 8, 11, 53, 103, 135, 159, 171, 175–6; global 8, 34, 165, 175
governance theory 10, 175
governance: global 4–5, 10–13, 25, 27, 32, 52, 173, 177–8; global health 68, 108–9, 114, 118, 122, 127; state-centred 12
government agencies 48, 115, 122, 140–1, 145, 169
GPGs *see* global public goods
GPPPHs *see* Global Public–Private Partnerships for Health
GPPPs (Global public–private partnerships) 27, 97, 119, 122

Hashemite Jordan Charity Organization (HAJCO) 131
Health Assembly 61–6, 68–9, 71, 74, 77, 90–1, 94, 96–7, 102–3, 105, 167; *see also* World Health Assembly
health for all 55–6, 82, 166, 170
healthcare 3, 82–3, 121, 123, 126–7, 136, 160, 162
healthcare sector 118–19, 134

HIV/AIDS 76, 109, 112–14, 120–2, 127, 152, 158
Hong Kong 1, 49, 51, 55, 58, 86, 89, 91, 105
human rights 16, 19–20, 29, 41, 49, 80, 82, 108, 116, 123, 135, 152, 166, 170–2, 175, 177
humanitarian action 5, 13, 17, 28, 30–4, 86
humanitarian aid projects 7, 119, 123, 129, 136
humanitarian arguments 59, 77, 89–90, 102
humanitarian assistance 4, 7, 31, 34, 114, 119, 123, 129, 143, 150–1, 162, 165, 168, 170
humanitarian interventions 29, 31–2, 171
humanitarian organizations 30, 32–3, 75, 125, 132, 145–6, 168, 170; Taiwanese 5, 75, 117, 123, 144–6, 168

iACT 116, 132
ICN (International Council of Nursing) 67, 75, 96
ICRC (International Committee of the Red Cross) 21, 30–1, 63, 65, 92
IGOs (international governmental organizations) 25, 27, 40–2, 94, 96, 115, 118, 121, 148; *see also* international organizations
IHRF (International Humanitarian Relief Fund) 114, 142
impartiality 20, 29, 33, 109
independence 29, 33, 46, 61, 66, 90, 93, 101, 103–5, 109, 152, 173, 175
Indian Ocean 129, 144, 151–3, 156, 158, 169, 174
infectious diseases 55, 60, 76, 84–5, 97, 109, 111, 113, 127–8, 158–9; outbreaks of 99–100; *see also* communicable diseases
Initiative on Public–Private Partnerships for Health (IPPPH) 122, 128
institutionalism 2, 11
integration theory 36
interactions, state–civil society 35, 68, 72
intergovernmental organizations 5, 40–1, 91–2, 118; *see also* IGOs
International Committee of the Red Cross *see* ICRC
International Council of Nursing *see* ICN
international governmental organizations *see* IGOs
international health cooperation 54–5, 95, 109
International Health Regulations 98–9, 108
international humanitarian law 29, 147
International Humanitarian Relief Fund (IHRF) 114, 142
International Non-Governmental Organizations (INGOs) 72–5, 97
international order 16, 38, 179
international organizations 38–40, 51, 94, 110, 114–15, 172; *see also* IGOs
International Paediatrics Association (IPA) 67, 75
International Pharmaceutical Federation (IPF) 67, 75, 96
International Society of Internal Medicine (ISIM) 126
IPA *see* International Paediatrics Association
IPF *see* International Pharmaceutical Federation
IPPPH (Initiative on Public–Private Partnerships for Health) 122, 128
Iraq 29, 125, 129, 131, 140, 144, 152, 169
ISIM (International Society of Internal Medicine) 126
Israel 15, 39, 42, 174

Kissinger 38–9
Kiwanis 117, 144
KMT 43–4, 91, 95, 137, 139, 147, 165, 169
Kosovo 29, 31, 59, 130–1, 156, 161, 175

League Health Organization 54
legitimacy 4–5, 10, 13–20, 25–6, 33–5, 175, 177
Liberia 39, 123, 125, 131, 139, 175
linking arrangements 2, 6–7, 19, 22, 27, 34, 68, 95, 117, 148, 151, 169, 176–7
loans 114, 121, 136, 138, 140, 142, 150–2, 162, 169; soft 119, 150
Love from Taiwan 125, 129, 140, 144, 152

Ma Ying-jeou 100, 104
Macedonia 123–4, 130, 132, 139, 156, 161
malaria 60, 76, 83–4, 109, 113, 122, 126, 149, 154–5, 159
Malawi 130, 146, 150–1, 155, 160–2, 165, 170, 172, 178
Malaysia 57, 85–6
market incentives 122, 159
market organizations 21, 25, 27, 30, 48, 96, 115, 144; Taiwanese 48–9, 67, 109, 141
material instruments 23, 119, 122, 125, 151, 169, 173, 177–8

material resources 16, 119, 121–2, 132, 139, 175, 177
medical aid programmes 125, 170–1; Taiwan's 69, 151
medical assistance 52, 115, 129, 132, 141, 144, 160, 166
medical cooperation 114, 155–6, 160; Taiwan's 34, 115, 150
medical journals 84, 155
medical missions 119, 130, 140, 145–6, 150, 153, 155, 160–2, 165
medical NGOs, Taiwanese 68, 96
medical professionals 56, 75, 94, 116
Medicines for Malaria Venture (MMV) 121, 128
Millennium: Declaration 108, 123, 137, 149, 158, 168; Development Goals 7, 123, 126, 133, 147, 149, 158–9
Ministry of Foreign Affairs *see* Taiwan Ministry of Foreign Affairs
MMV *see* Medicines for Malaria Venture
Mongolian and Tibetan Affairs Commission 143
multilateral organizations 16, 160
multinational corporations 25–6, 111, 114

neutrality 20, 29, 33, 109
NGOs (non-governmental organizations) 26–7, 31–3, 49–51, 72–4, 77–8, 92–3, 95–7, 113, 122–6, 140–1, 151–3, 163, 169–70, 172–4; Taiwanese 4, 6–7, 49–50, 95–6, 111, 115, 124–5, 132–3, 140, 146, 152, 156, 163, 174
non-profit organizations *see* NPOs
non-state organizations 6, 18–19, 36, 40, 47, 51, 64, 80, 96, 121, 123, 172; Taiwanese 6, 51, 67, 95, 115, 132, 166, 173
norm-setting 2, 18, 26, 34, 94, 113, 168
norms: aid 110, 134, 136; economic 7, 107, 111, 137–9; global 7–8, 28, 34, 112, 163, 165, 168, 174; humanitarian 6, 56, 84, 107, 109, 136; medical 6–137
NPOs (non-profit organizations) 21, 47–8, 51, 64, 73, 95, 142, 145; Taiwanese 47

observer status 6, 53–4, 61–3, 66–8, 70–1, 75–7, 80, 84–5, 89, 91–4, 97, 101–5, 172
ODA (Official Development Assistance) 111, 114, 117, 121, 126, 129, 137–8, 151–3, 156–7, 161, 169; Taiwan's 140, 150, 153
OECD 108, 112, 118–19, 126, 129, 137, 140, 151–3, 156, 158, 160–1, 173
Office International d'Hygiène Publique (OIHP) 54
Official Development Assistance *see* ODA
outbreaks 57–8, 78, 85, 90, 97, 99; *see also* epidemic outbreaks
Overseas Taiwanese 51, 68, 120
Overseas Taiwanese organizations 96

Palestine 63, 81, 92–3, 175
pharmaceutical companies 94, 96–7, 109, 113, 122, 128, 134, 159
Pintung Christian Hospital 115, 133, 146, 150, 153
policy instruments 6–7, 11–12, 19, 23–4, 34, 36, 68, 79–80, 93, 95, 117, 151, 165–70, 174, 177
policy tools 2, 19, 22–3
polio 56, 60, 84, 127
polio eradication campaign 121, 123, 144, 148–9, 153, 155, 161, 169
political systems theory 2, 11
poverty 60, 111–12, 120
protection 20, 28, 31–2, 138
public health 17, 55, 60, 63, 73, 76, 78, 83, 108, 146, 159
public health emergency 157, 167–8
public health experts 78, 88

quasi-permanent observer status 98, 104–5

recipients 24, 109–10, 137–8, 140–1; *see also* aid recipient countries
recognition 1, 12, 14–16, 133, 149, 163, 167, 170–1, 173; global 40, 108, 136, 166, 170, 172, 174
Red Cross 25, 28, 63, 65, 76–7, 90, 117, 124, 147
refugees 32–3, 113, 116–17, 123–4, 130–2, 156, 161
regime theory 2, 11
Republic of China 15, 35–40, 42–5, 59, 69–70, 75, 78, 81–3, 91, 93, 97–8, 101–2, 166
Republic of Korea 81
République Centrafricaine 69
reunification 16, 36, 46, 49, 104
Rotary Club 144, 161
Rotary International 75, 121, 123, 144, 148, 169

São Tomé and Príncipe 39, 130, 154–5

SARS 57–8, 71, 76, 86–90, 97, 99, 103, 129, 167
Security Council 30–1, 38–9, 82, 136, 139–40, 167, 171, 173
Senegal 39, 69, 138–40
Singapore 1, 55, 58, 83, 86
smallpox 60, 83–4, 109, 127
South Africa 15, 39, 70, 81, 93, 174
Southeast Asia 48–9, 65, 116, 144, 173
sovereign 13, 77, 166, 177
Sovereign Order of Malta 15–16, 63, 92–3
sovereignty 3, 14–16, 20, 35–6, 41, 55, 69, 80, 89, 166, 171–2, 177; China's 37, 168, 172
State Department 70, 98, 102
state organizations 22, 25, 31, 114, 125, 141, 168
state–society interactions 43, 47
state–society relations 5, 46
state-to-state interactions 68, 95
statehood 5, 35–6, 81, 89, 175
statehood claims 92, 175
states: aspiring 16, 171, 175; authoritarian 43–4; donor 114, 135; independent 14, 36, 41, 104; irregular 1, 6, 8, 34–5, 53, 165, 171, 173–4; isolated 16; recognized 41, 171; regular 16, 166, 168, 171, 173; sovereign 14, 92, 106; strong 44
supplementary item 69, 96
symbolic instruments 23, 125, 135, 152, 170, 178

Taipei 38, 41, 66, 87–8, 101, 126, 138, 140, 143, 160
Taiwan CDC 58, 129
Taiwan Government Information Office 75, 100
Taiwan International Health Action 126, 156, 192
Taiwan International Medical Alliance (TIMA) 5, 68, 115–17, 124, 132, 146–7
Taiwan Ministry of Foreign Affairs 7, 49–51, 55–6, 59, 66, 77, 104, 114–15, 119, 123–6, 130–3, 145–6, 148–51, 161–2
Taiwan–Mongolia Association 143, 173
Taiwan Red Cross 86, 90, 109, 117, 124–5, 132, 147
Taiwan Roots Medical Peace Corps *see* TRMPC
Taiwan–Russia Association 143, 155
Taiwan Straits 36, 42, 101, 147, 181, 186–8
Taiwan–Tibet Exchange Foundation 143–4
Taiwan's health authorities 59, 83, 85; *see also* Department of Health
Taiwan's status 7, 41, 49, 95, 100–1, 107, 144, 149, 151–2, 161, 171
Taiwan-based organizations 107, 174
Taiwanese businessmen 115, 120, 144, 173
Taiwanese journalists 41–2, 104, 166
TaiwanICDF 7, 108, 112, 114–15, 119, 123–4, 129–30, 138, 140–3, 146, 150–1, 153, 155, 160, 172
TaiwanIHA 126, 129, 132, 148, 152–3, 169
TANs *see* Transnational advocacy networks
TB 109, 113, 122, 155, 159
TDR (Tropical Disease Research) 91, 118, 148, 167
Tibetan Government-in-exile 143–4
TIMA *see* Taiwan International Medical Alliance
Transnational advocacy networks (TAN) 27
transparency 16, 72–3, 77, 108, 123, 135, 140, 168–9
TRIPS (Trade-related aspects of Intellectual Property) 113, 157, 159
TRMPC (Taiwan Roots Medical Peace Corps) 116, 125–6, 131–3, 145, 156
Tropical Disease Research *see* TDR
Tzu Chi 50, 86, 115–16, 119–20, 123–6, 131–3, 146, 151–2, 156, 163, 168

UNAIDS 76, 94, 97, 113, 118, 121–3, 127, 148, 170
UNHCR 30–1, 65, 113, 118, 124, 150, 160
UNICEF 30–1, 65, 76, 84, 86, 112–13, 118, 121, 126–7, 146, 148, 150, 154, 157
United Nations Economic and Social Council 113, 163
United States 32, 38, 41–2, 71, 83, 86, 92, 128, 173
universality 20, 35, 60, 80–1, 109, 166
UNOCHA 31, 58, 86
UNPO (Unrepresented Nations and Peoples Organization) 41, 172

Vatican 16, 40, 63, 77, 160
Vietnam 36–7, 55, 58–9, 87, 117, 146
visibility 8, 97, 149, 152, 154, 161, 164–5, 169–71

warlords 14–16, 178
WFP (World Food Programme) 30–1, 118, 150

WHA *see* World Health Assembly
WHO campaign, Taiwan's 1, 4, 6, 49, 53, 61, 65, 67–8, 76–7, 80, 100, 166
WHO collaborating center 65, 87–8, 100
WHPA (World Health Professionals Alliance) 96
WMA *see* World Medical Association
World Bank 10, 40, 76, 91, 94, 113, 118–19, 126–8, 148, 157, 160, 170
World Health Assembly (WHA) 4, 7, 41, 53, 66–73, 75, 77–9, 81–2, 84–5, 88–9, 93–6, 100–2, 104, 166–8
World Health Organization 4, 6, 42, 53–4, 61–2, 66, 82, 94, 100, 104, 108, 113, 121, 162
World Health Professionals Alliance (WHPA) 96
World Medical Association (WMA) 67–8, 71, 75, 96
World Vision Taiwan 117, 121, 124, 126, 132, 134
WTO (World Trade Organization) 40, 42, 92–3, 101, 157, 172

For Product Safety Concerns and Information please contact our EU representative GPSR@taylorandfrancis.com
Taylor & Francis Verlag GmbH, Kaufingerstraße 24, 80331 München, Germany

www.ingramcontent.com/pod-product-compliance
Lightning Source LLC
LaVergne TN
LVHW011129300926
849160LV00008B/571